I0120891

Table of Contents

The Skillful Questioner

Problems cannot be solved by the same level of thinking that created them.
~ Albert Einstein

During the Renaissance there was a massive resurgence of learning and a gradual yet widespread shift in education, leading to economic growth and development, political and social reform, and an increase in trade and commerce.

The Industrial Revolution was a major turning point in human history. There were immense technological advancements, economic progress, income & population growth, and an increase in the standard of living never seen before.

Why?

They were asking themselves powerful questions that shifted the way they approached problems, and spurred curiosity and creativity.

Today, we are on the verge of another major shift. To make the leap we need to make we must ask ourselves and our clients questions that achieve & surpass that same level of curiosity and creativity.

The quality of questions we ask directly influence the knowledge we acquire and the actions we take.

By asking quality, empowering questions we can find the answers leading to the change we seek.

Being a skillful questioner is more than just the words used in the questions. It's as much about how you ask the questions as it is about the words you use. Having no attachment to the outcome of the question and addressing the questioner with curiosity, objectivity and in a non-confrontational manner creates an atmosphere of safety for the questionee to answer honestly and thoroughly.

With over 30 years of coaching, training, facilitation, and experiential learning experience between the two of them, both Denny & Kathy Jo recognize even the most skilled professionals can sometimes get stuck finding the right questions.

Asking powerful questions allow the questionee to see things differently, open up creativity, gain new perspectives, see solutions, discover their own answers, deepens relationships and trust, and improves problem-solving and decision-making abilities.

You can ask the most empowering questions and unlock amazing possibilities, but unless you truly listen and the questionee feels that intent, forward movement is stunted. Listening is an important part of communication as is asking powerful questions. However, not all listening is effective listening.

It is said that hearing is a physical ability. We all hear. We don't always listen. Listening is a skill, one that must be practiced and intentional to be effective.

As a vital part of the questioning process, listening enables:
- The acquisition of new information
- Greater insight to the values, strengths, behavior and needs of the questionee
- The questionee to discover his / her own perspectives of the situation
- Trust & Rapport
- Understanding of underlying meaning
- Motivation
- Depth & Intimacy
- Mutual understanding
- The questionee to feel heard and understood

Levels of Listening

There are 4 Levels of Listening. We have all experienced listening to others and being listened to at each level. The higher the level the more energy is required to maintain that level. Not every conversation you have will take place at the Intuitive Listening level.

1. **Competitive Listening**: The main focus in Competitive Listening is on the listener's own thoughts. Here the listener is more interested in their own views and is waiting for an opportunity to jump in and react.

2. **Attentive Listening**: The main focus in Attentive Listening is on the words being said. There is genuine interest in hearing and understanding what is being said but assumes an understanding, not checking with the questionee for confirmation.

3. **Reflective Listening**: The main focus in Reflective Listening is on a deeper and clarified understanding of what is being said. There is genuine interest in listening, not just hearing, as well as understanding what is being said and confirms that understanding, often through mirroring back the exact information shared.

4. **Intuitive Listening**: The main focus in Intuitive Listening is an understanding of the meaning behind what is said. There is genuine desire to understand not only the meaning of what is being said but also the tone, pitch, speed, of what's being said, the body language that accompanies the words, what is being said behind the words, and what is NOT being said.

We all know how important communication is. However, the vast majority of communication isn't spoken. According to studies done in the '70s by Albert Mehrabian, only 7% of communication takes place through exchange of words. The remaining 93% of information is communicated through body language, eye contact, and pitch, speed, tone and volume of the voice.

Understanding that most information is not communicated through words, to be a powerful listener there are several things you have to keep in mind while listening to the questionee.

Keys to Powerful Listening

1. Intentions are set to gain a greater understanding of the questionee, their behavior, thinking, values, beliefs, perspectives and needs.
2. Stay Curious.
3. Detached Involvement: the ability to tap into deep levels of empathy and place yourself in the questionees position, understanding their thoughts and feelings without taking on their emotions.
4. Focus on what is being communicated in all areas – body language, tone, pace, pitch, energy – while not focusing on your response.
5. Offer feedback and request clarification if necessary.
6. Remember silence is golden. Don't be afraid of silence. Allow the questionee to sit with the question and ponder.
7. Use Intuitive Listening as much as possible.

When entering a conversation where you are required to deeply listen and understand questionees, try your best to enter the situation with as much energy as possible.

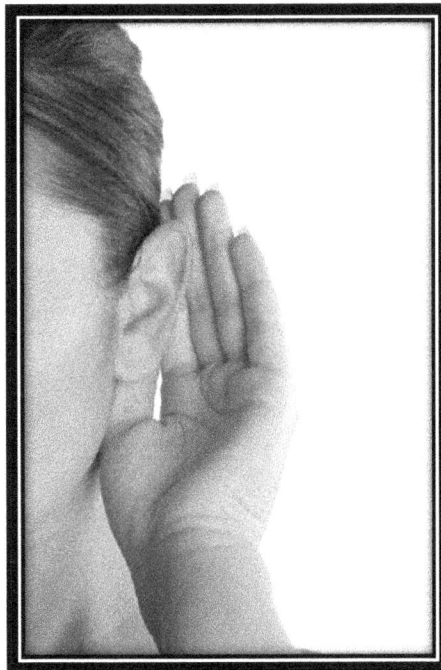

Powerful Questions + Intuitive Listening + Acknowledgement + Time to Respond = Unlocked Potential & Possibilities

Making Questions Powerful

Asking the right questions in the right way is key to achieving the right results. Powerful questions immediately access our creative, holistic brain from which solutions are born. These thought provoking questions are designed to forward your client's actions through clarifying, inspiring, probing, challenging, affirming, exploring, opening new possibilities, connecting, assessing, and evaluating, leading to the right solutions for your client.

When crafting questions, there are 3 things you must consider.
1. The Scope of the Question
2. The Construction of the Question
3. Assumptions & Bias in the Question

Scope

The Scope is defined as the range or subject matter that something deals with or to which it is relevant. The scope covers the domain of inquiry. Matching the scope of the question to meet the needs of inquiry increases the capacity to effect change and sets the questionee up for success. Therefore, keep within realistic boundaries of the situation and questionee's knowledge and power.

For example: "How can you best change your perspective?" as opposed to "How can you change the perspective within the organization?"

When determining the scope of your question you must first determine the scope of the answer you are seeking. If you are looking for greater clarification you must ask questions designed to gain clarity. If you are looking for greater insight, you must ask questions designed to go deeper. If you are looking at obstacles you must ask questions designed to uncover blocks. The scope of the answer determines the category of the question to achieve an appropriate response. You can find the question categories under the General Questions section of this book.

Construction

The construction of a question consists of the language, intention and tone you take when asking the question. A question's construction is a critical element in either opening up one's mind to possibilities or closing the mind to solutions. The construction of a question can determine the depth and direction of the answers. Are you looking for a direct yes or no answer? Ask a closed-ended question. Are you looking for deeper clarification? Do you want to open choices or create a new picture? Ask open-ended questions.

The construction of a question stimulates reflective thinking and deepens the conversation. Starting your question with either "who" or "how" determines the level and direction of inquiry. For example: "Who can help you to make this happen?" "How can this happen?"

When constructing the question, ask yourself what "work" you want this question to do.

Assumptions and Bias

Part of being human is that our experiences and perspectives influence the way we think. We all carry with us assumptions and biases. We cannot eliminate them. Awareness of assumptions and biases allow us to be on the look-out for them as we construct and ask our questions, and listen to the answer.

One of the most commonly used questions containing an assumption or bias is "What is wrong?" This question assumes a negative.

Reframing is a potent way to reword questions freeing them of assumptions and bias such as from "What's wrong?" to "What happened?" Reframing encourages deeper reflection and shifts assumptions into possibilities for creating forward action.

A Word About "Why"

Some of the most powerful questions begin with "Why." Some of the most dangerous questions begin with "Why."

Why-questions can lead to greater insight and more thorough answers.

They ask the questionee to go deeper and evaluate. Answers to why-questions speak about the inner feelings, beliefs, and motives of the questionee. Because of the highly personal nature of why-questions safety and trust must be established in the relationship. If not, a why-question can easily trigger reactive behaviors and blame leading detracting from solutions.

The difference between getting greater insight and triggering reaction is the level of safety the questionee feels in the relationship and the way in which the question is asked.

If safety and trust have been established on both sides of the relationship and a why-question is the most appropriate question to ask, stay curious when asking your question. This will keep the non-verbal elements of asking a question as well as your intention on maintaining safety and trust and away from blame.

Choose why-questions carefully and sparingly.

Characteristics of a Powerful Question

1. Solutions-focused
2. Clear & Simple
3. Involves Values & Ideals
4. Generates Curiosity
5. Stimulates Reflection
6. Thought-Provoking
7. Engages Attention
8. Focused
9. Touches Deeper Meaning
10. Leads to More Questions

How to Use This Book

As you encounter a specific challenge around Wellness in your life or your client's life, you may become stuck and not know where to go next. This book is designed to assist in getting you and your clients unstuck by sparking new, unique, and in-depth questions. Use these questions as is or allow them to inspire new ideas for you.

Open / Closed-Ended Questions Chart: Open-Ended questions are designed to require the answerer to go deeper and give more detail. These types of questions should be used as often as possible to gain greater detail, inquiry, and increase understanding. Closed-Ended questions are excellent for commitment. These are used ONLY when looking for a "yes" or "no" response.

General Wellness Questions: These general Wellness-based questions are a great starting point for coaching around health & wellness issues. These questions are designed around a basic coaching approach of: clarifying, creating a vision, defining choice, identifying blocks and barriers, evaluating, prioritizing, probing, and scaling. Use these questions as touchstones throughout the process. Categorized based on your client's specific needs and situation, these questions increase the scope of the coaching relationship.

Wellness Wheel: The Wellness Wheel is a self-awareness assessment you can use for yourself or your client to rate the level of satisfaction in each area of Health & Wellness. Use this wheel to broaden the scope of coaching to encompass each area and create their ideal health.

Wheel Specific Questions: As your coaching partnership deepens and gaps in wellness skills present themselves, target different areas of Health & Wellness more thoroughly through these questions. Use these Wheel Specific Question to prolong the coaching partnership and develop more consciousness around health.

Wellness Values / Qualities Assessment: Rating Wellness Values / Qualities by how important they are to you or your client, and how much you walk your talk can help you identify where gaps may be in Health & Wellness Skills. This is an excellent resource in identifying areas and opportunities for growth.

Blank Wheel: Using the Blank Wheel, fill in your or your client's top 8 Wellness Values / Qualities and rank these to address the gaps of creating their ideal health. You can also develop new coaching assignments and opportunities around each area.

Wellness Quotes: This collection of Wellness Quotes is a great resource for either your own marketing efforts or to deepen the level of thinking for your clients. Use these quotes to send inspirational emails, add to your website, use as topics for your newsletters or to Tweet.

SMART Goals Checklist: SMART Goals help ensure success. Goals that are unattainable or unreasonable are a direct line to failure. Failure stifles excitement, passion, and commitment. To ensure the success of your clients, check each goal against the SMART Goals checklist to determine how viable the goal truly is and keep your client's on track.

Additional Uses for This Book

Coaching/Consulting Role

→ Use the Wellness Wheel Assessment in a Complementary Session

→ Assess a client's level of satisfaction in the 8 key areas of the Wellness Wheel in an introductory session to establish the partnership foundation

→ Use SMART Goals checklist as an evaluation & progression tool

→ Create accountability around the SMART Goals checklist

→ Identify strengths & gaps in each area of the Wellness Wheel

→ Identify initial coaching goals

→ Use the questions as preparation for coaching sessions

→ Create customized assignments using the questions

→ Create visualizations & meditations based around the Wellness Wheel segments or Questions

→ Use quotes in sessions to stimulate fresh perspectives

→ Add quotes to client emails for inspiration

→ Create a customized assignment by journaling on quotes

→ Create a mastermind or group discussion around a specific quote

→ Help clients set goals using the SMART Goals checklist

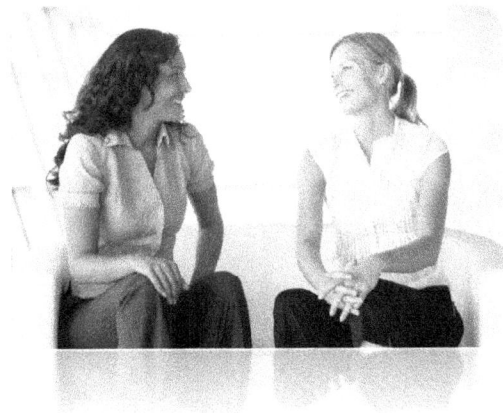

Product & Services Development

→   Use this book and the Wellness Wheel as your Signature Program

→   Use Wellness Wheel Assessment in a workshop as an assessment or discussion tool

→   Add Wellness Wheel Assessment to your current Signature Program or product

→   Use questions as an idea generator

→   Create an E-course / E-book / E-workbook series around segments of the Wellness Wheel

→   Develop workshops & seminars around segments of the Wellness Wheel

→   Form Mastermind Groups around key Wellness Wheel segments

→   Use Wellness Values / Qualities list as an idea generator

→   Write an E-course / E-book / E-workbook on a grouping of Wellness Values

→   Create Workshops & Seminars on a grouping of Wellness Values

→   Add a quote to a product for inspiration or point emphasis

→   Use quote in workshop as a discussion topic

→   Use SMART Goals checklist in a workshop as tool to move participants forward

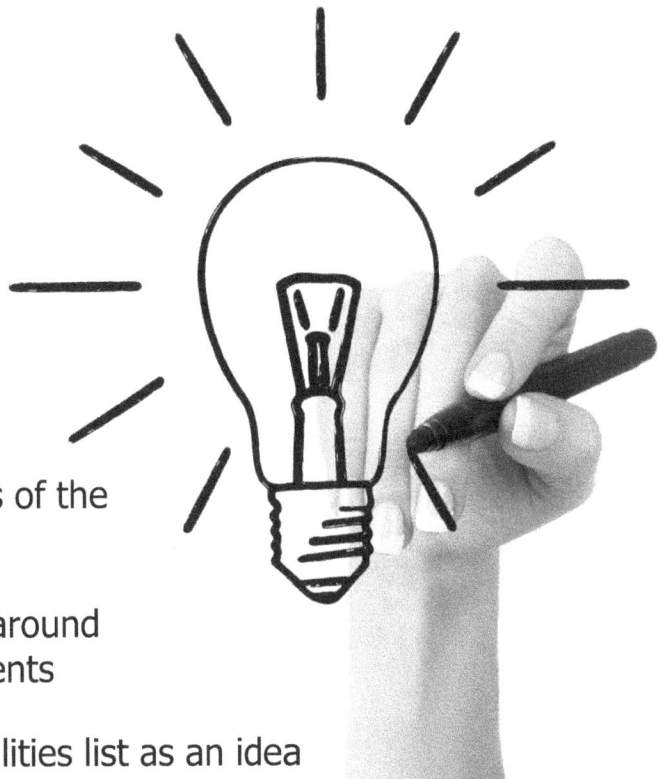

Marketing / Business Development

→ Use Wellness Wheel Assessment as a prospect pre-qualifier

→ Create a prequalifying survey for prospects with questions

→ Use questions or quotes in ezine / newsletter

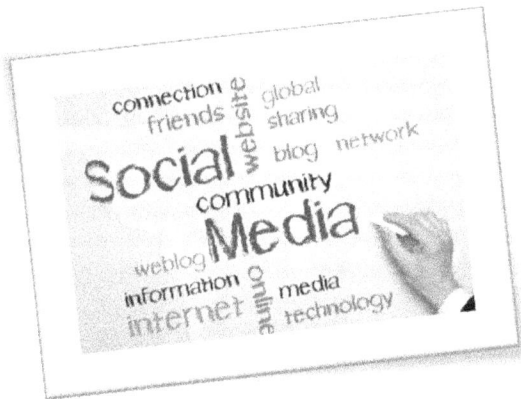

→ Post a question / quote to your target audience on a LinkedIn Discussion

→ Use a series of questions to outline a promotional teleclass

→ Create a free download of questions around a particular topic

→ Use questions in Blog & Twitter Posts

→ Write an article based on the questions

→ Write an article based on an individual Wellness Value

→ Use the Wellness Values Assessment as a pre-coaching prep form

→ Create an ezine / newsletter around individual Wellness Value

→ Post a quote on your blog / Facebook / LinkedIn asking for comments about how it relates to the topic

→ Use a quote to inspire a podcast or video

→ Use quote to motivate an article idea

→ Post Quote on Blog / Twitter

Open-Ended vs. Closed-Ended Questions

Open-Ended questions invite others to discuss in detail what is important to them. They are used to gather information, establish rapport, and increase understanding. These questions do not lead and are not geared towards expected outcomes. When used, the asker must be willing to listen and respond appropriately.

Closed-Ended questions are used to elicit a definitive answer. Use only when you want a definite yes or no. They are particularly useful when gaining a commitment.

Ask Open-Ended questions whenever possible.

Open-Ended Questions Start with:	Closed-Ended Questions Start with:
Who	Is
What	Does
How	Are
Why	Do
When	Will
Where	Can

General Wellness Questions

Clarifying

Clarifying questions are designed to lay the groundwork and foundation for attaining goals. They set the stage, remove ambiguity, elicit details, and supply known facts.

Ask Clarifying Questions when you need a clear picture of where the questionee is currently at, what resources are available, what perspectives they have, as well as want a picture of where the questionee is coming from, what they want, and the reality of the situation.

Ask these questions as a starting point, to establish a framework.

Example of Clarifying Questions

Questionee: I want to feel more freedom in my life.

Questioner: What do you mean by more freedom?

Questionee: I mean to have the ability to do what I want when I want to.

Questioner: Give me an example.

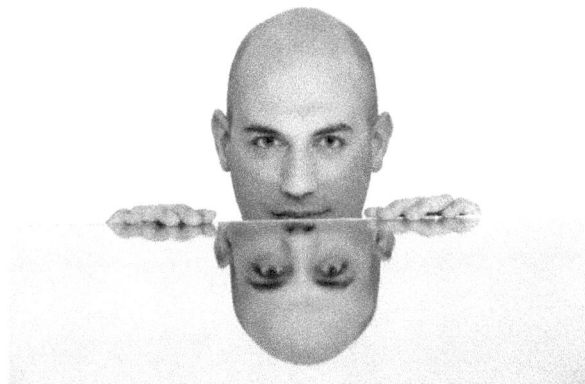

Clarifying Questions

→ Who has impacted your overall health and wellness?

→ Who has encouraged you to be healthier?

→ Who has inspired you to adopt a healthier lifestyle?

→ Who is the healthiest person you know?

→ Who stresses you out?

→ Who grounds you?

→ What is health?

→ What is wellness?

→ What does wellness mean to you?

→ What makes a healthy person?

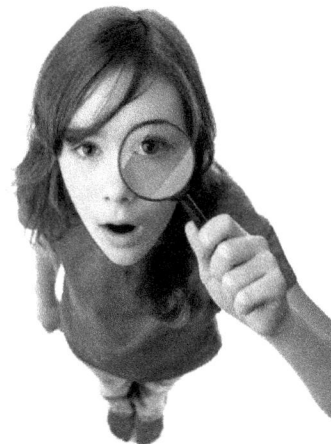

→ What do healthy people do?

→ What does a healthy person look like?

→ What do you most want to change?

→ What is your biggest health concern?

→ What is your greatest hope?

→ What would a health-conscious person do?

→ What should a health-conscious person avoid?

→ If your current state of health were described with one word, what would that be?

→ Where in your life do you need a greater sense of wellness?

→ Where have you sought out help in the past?

→ Where could you begin to make the changes you desire?

→ Where do you like to go to unwind?

→ Where is your body guiding you to go?

→ When was the first time you became aware your health was not where you wanted it to be?

→ When are you at your best?

→ When are you at your worst?

→ Why have you decided to make your health a priority?

→ Why is feeling healthier important for you?

→ Why are you seeking help now?

→ How do you express your wellness?

→ How do you stay healthy?

→ How do you define wellness?

→ How do you want your body to feel?

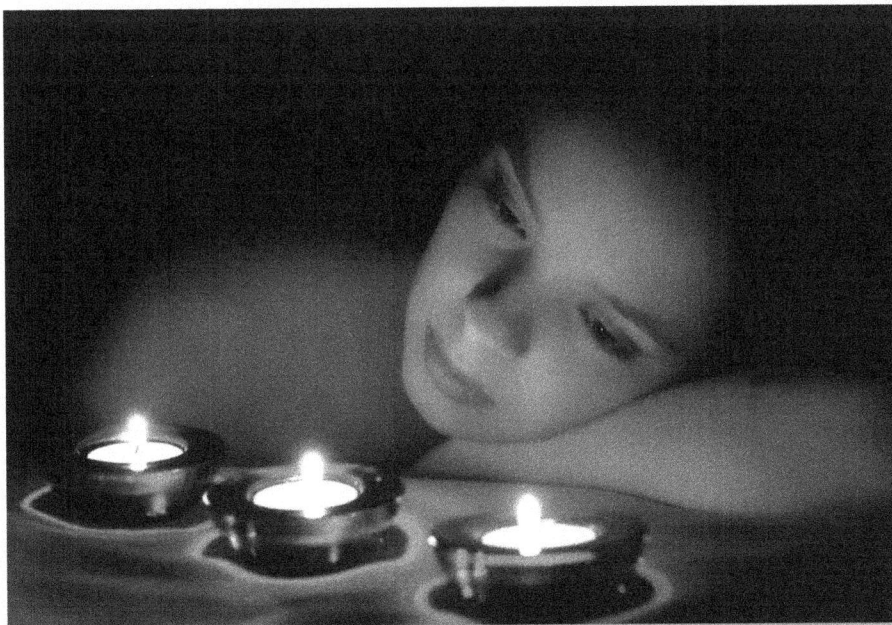

Visioning

Visioning questions are designed to establish a desired end result. These questions create a picture of the future so a plan on how to get there can be created.

Visioning Questions allow the questionee to "see" the result they are working to achieve. This opens possibilities, engages creativity, and keeps motivation high and direction clear.

Ask Visioning Questions when creating a new reality, establishing an end-result, identifying the ideal, or giving direction to move forward.

Example of Visioning Questions

Questioner: What would you ideally like to see happen?

Questionee: I would like to move to the country away from the noise and congestion of the city. I would like to grow my own food, and live more simply. I would like to see the stars at night and hear the crickets sing.

Questioner: In this ideal vision, what do you see yourself doing?

Questionee: I see myself writing that book I keep talking about and having time to putter around in my flower garden.

Questioner: How would you feel if you had that?

Questionee: I see myself really happy, living a good life with the people I love, enjoying the things that give my life meaning.

Questioner: That is a beautiful picture for you.

Questionee: Yes it is!

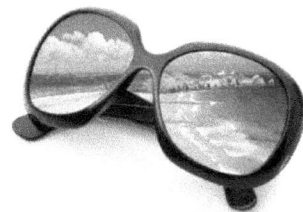

Visioning Questions

→ Who would you like to model your wellness lifestyle after?

→ Who do you imagine you can become?

→ Who will you be in a year's time?

→ Who is the ideal you?

→ What does an unhealthy lifestyle look like?

→ What would you change about your overall wellness?

→ What difference would having a healthier life mean to you?

→ What type of lifestyle do you want?

→ What is your ideal body type?

→ What would life be like as a healthy person?

→ What does wellness mean?

→ Where do you see your health in 3 months / 6 months / a year?

→ Where would be your ideal relaxation area?

→ Where could a healthy vibrant body take you?

→ Where will you be in 3 months / 6 months / a year if nothing changes?

→ Where do you see yourself right now?

→ When you achieve the type of well-being you seek, what will be different?

→ When you are at your optimal wellness, what will you be able to do?

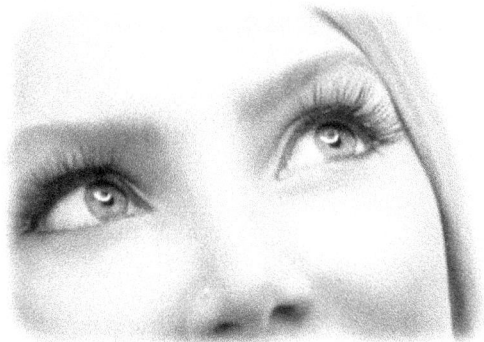

→ When you are 70 years old, what would you like to be able to do?

→ Why would you imagine anything less for yourself?

→ Why is it important to envision a healthier you?

→ Why do you imagine that?

→ Why is holding a healthier vision for your life essential?

→ Why do you want to be healthier?

→ How will your day to day actions be different as a completely healthy person?

→ How would you like to live?

→ How could you be healthier?

→ How grand is your vision of wellness?

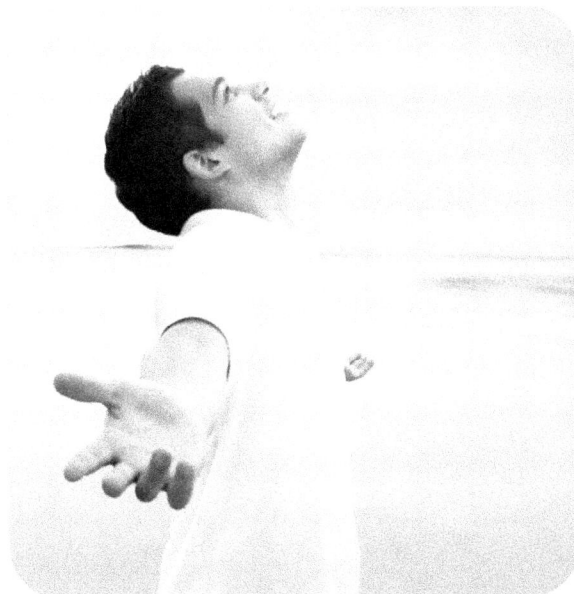

Choice

Choice Questions are meant to show options, empower, and accept responsibility. These questions lend to out-of-the-box thinking and demonstrate options and opportunities.

Ask Choice Questions when questionee feels trapped, hopeless, or feels as though there is no other answer, and needs a new perspective & empowerment to move forward.

Example of Choice Question

Questionee: I don't know what to do. I really would like to attend that seminar next Saturday and Sunday but my husband wants to take the kids to the cabin that same weekend. We always do everything together.

Questioner: If you knew no-one would be upset, what options do you have to resolve this?

Questionee: You mean, if I went to the seminar and my husband took the boys to the cabin without me?

Questioner: What would happen if that could be the reality?

Questionee: Well that certainly would be different. Maybe that would work. I will talk with my husband tonight.

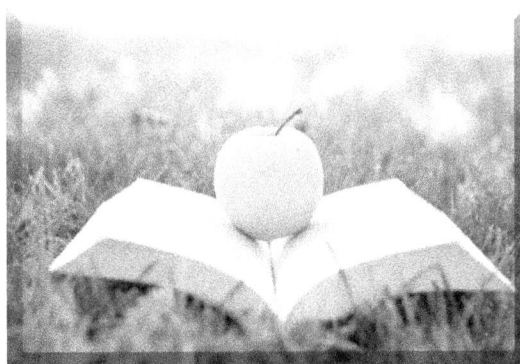

Choice Questions

→ Who supports your choices?

→ Who can help you decide what is best?

→ What drives your healthy life-style?

→ What drives your unhealthy life-style?

→ What are your choices?

→ What decisions do you need to make?

→ What would be the healthiest choice?

→ What is yours to do?

→ What healthy options do you have currently available to you?

→ What is your favorite way to exercise?

→ What is the best choice for you?

→ Where is the best place to begin?

→ Where have you made the healthiest choices in the past?

→ Where are you good at making healthy choices now?

→ Where is there a discrepancy?

→ When does stress influence your eating / exercising / sleeping habits?

→ When is wellness a choice and when is it a consequence?

→ When faced with a healthy choice / unhealthy choice, when do you choose the healthy / unhealthy choice?

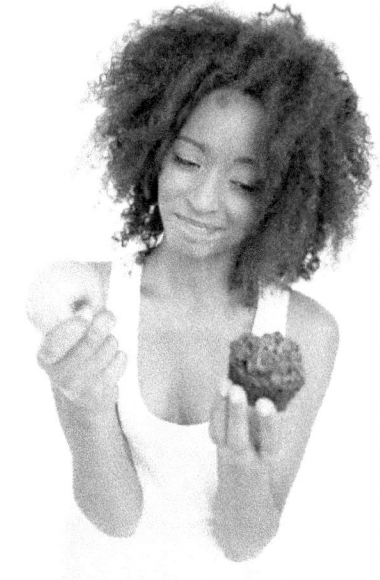

→ When would you like to get started with that plan?

→ Why is having a healthy body necessary?

→ Why would you do that knowing it is unhealthy for you?

→ Why not make that choice now?

→ Why would you do anything that negatively impacts your sense of wellness?

→ How soon will you begin?

→ How often do you make healthy decisions regarding your well-being?

→ How often do you talk yourself out of a healthier option?

→ How can you get clear on all your choices?

→ If you were to think of your body as your business, as your car, as your favorite shoes, as one of your children, etc. how would you treat it then?

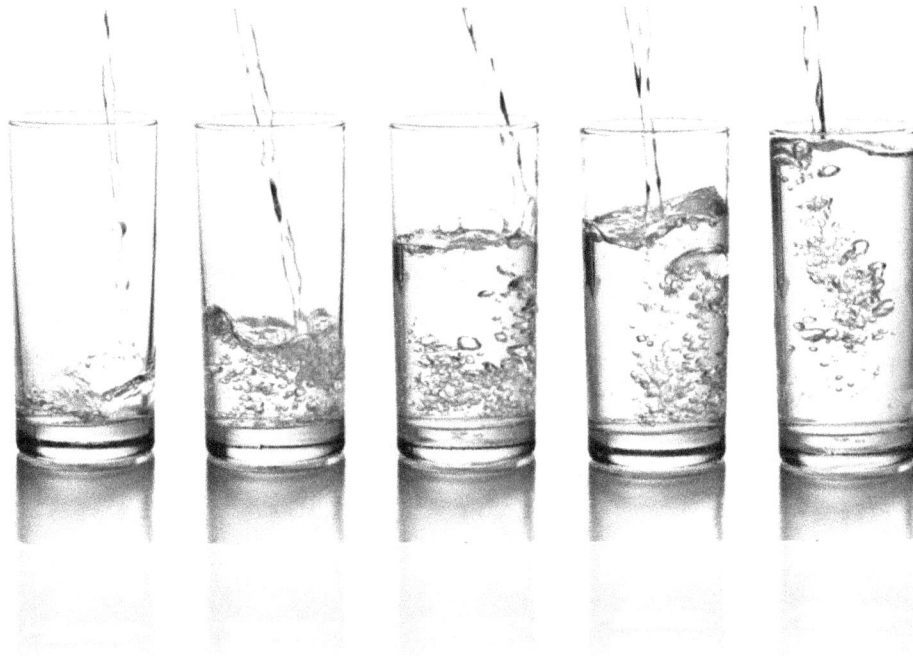

Blocks & Barriers

These questions are designed to uncover & examine what is stopping the questionee from moving forward, seeing progress, and gaining what they truly want.

Ask Blocks and Barrier Questions when you sense hesitation, resistance, goal hopping, or a belief they are unable to move forward.

Example of Blocks & Barriers Questions

Questionee: I really would like to date again but can't seem to put myself out there.

Questioner: What do you think is getting in the way?

Questionee: I'm not sure.....maybe my fear.

Questioner: Fear of what?

Questionee: Fear of not being attractive enough....of no one being interested in me.

Questioner: So you would rather stay home alone where it is safe than risk getting rejected again.

Questionee: As pitiful as that sounds, yes, I think that is it.

Questioner: How well will that work for you?

Questionee: Not very well at all since I want to meet someone! I guess we have some more work to do!

Questioner: I guess we do!

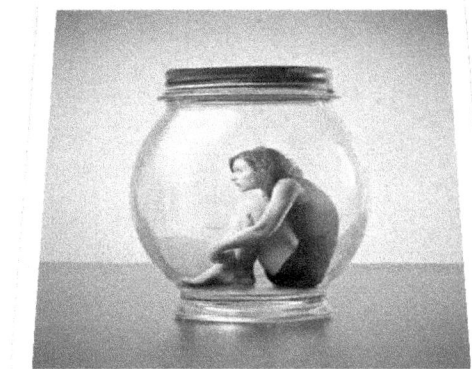

Blocks & Barriers Questions

→ Who has undermined your overall wellness?

→ Who would you be if nothing changed?

→ Who sabotages your wellness efforts?

→ What internal or external blocks do you have that hold you back from creating a healthy life?

→ What keeps you up at night?

→ What weighs you down?

→ What does your inner-critic say to you when you eat / don't exercise / make unhealthy choices?

→ What is the strongest influence you feel keeping you tethered to an unhealthy life?

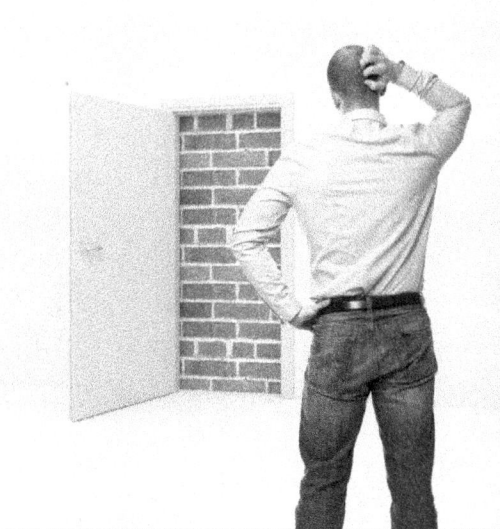

→ What is your biggest wellness challenge today?

→ What assumptions are you making about your wellness?

→ What makes that challenge particularly difficult?

→ What would happen if that issue persisted?

→ What is the hardest thing about living well?

→ What do you most want to overcome?

→ What does this block look like? Feel like? Sound like?

→ What assumptions are you making about your wellness?

→ Where do you sabotage your own well-being?

→ Where do you want to get to?

→ Where do you feel the greatest obstacle lies, in your mind, body, or soul?

→ Where to do stumble over your best made plans?

→ Where to do feel stuck in your body?

→ Where do your beliefs about who you are limit your wellness goals?

→ When do you feel the most blocked?

→ When do you feel the most free?

→ When was the last time you were able to overcome a big obstacle?

→ When do you feel the healthiest?

→ When do you feel the unhealthiest?

→ When are you on top of the world?

→ Why haven't you been able to do that in the past?

→ Why don't you want to change?

→ Why is your wellness taking a back seat?

→ Why are you letting that stop you?

→ Why do you need to get through this?

→ How have you been able to successfully move past obstacles in the past?

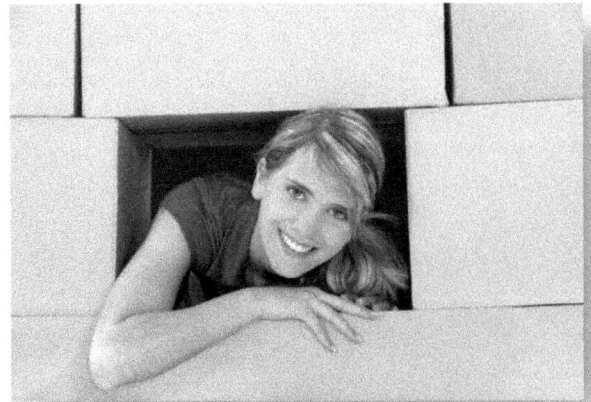

→ How could you use those strategies / skills / beliefs now to move you forward?

→ How much do you want to make these changes?

→ How does staying the same help you? Hurt you?

→ How does the media influence your thoughts about what is truly healthy?

→ How has your interpretation of wellness affected your health?

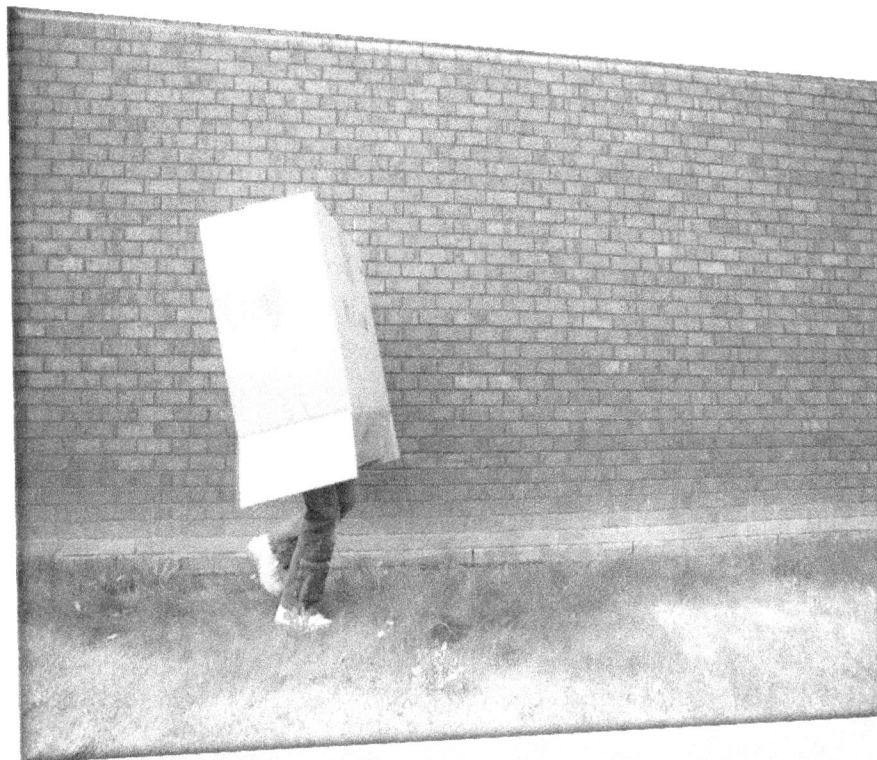

Evaluating

Evaluating Questions determine criteria. They evaluate or estimate the nature, quality, extent or significance of situations. They assess factors such as needs, issues, processes, performance, and outcomes. They can also determine the pros & cons of a situation.

Ask Evaluating Questions when the questionee needs to establish a clearer sense of their wants and needs related to a particular situation.

Example of Evaluating Questions

Questionee: I want to achieve more success at work.

Questioner: What would that look like?

Questionee: I would work more efficiently and get things done on time.

Questioner: What would be different if you were more efficient?

Questionee: I would lead meetings with more confidence and get more buy-in from the team.

Questioner: How would it feel if you achieved all of that?

Questionee: Great!

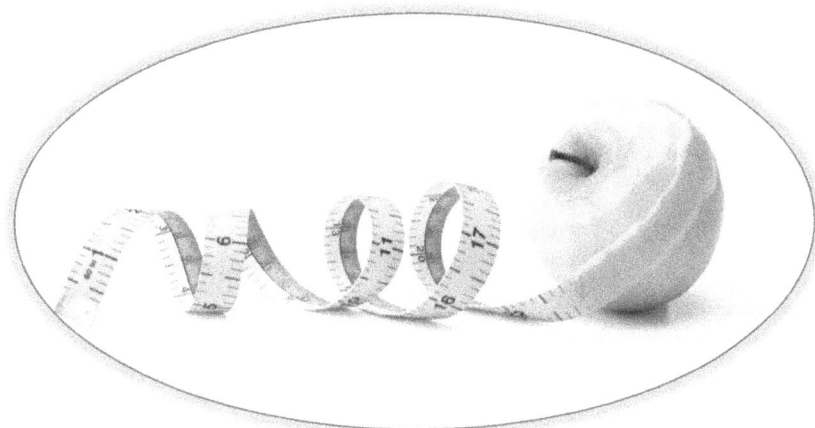

Evaluating Questions

→ Who do you know with a healthy lifestyle?

→ Who do you know with an unhealthy lifestyle?

→ What does wellness look like as a youth?

→ What does wellness look like as an adult?

→ What does wellness look like in old age?

→ What kind of wellness program would work best for you?

→ What is the hardest thing about maintaining a healthy lifestyle?

→ What is the easiest thing about maintaining a healthy lifestyle?

→ Where do you feel the healthiest in your life right now?

→ Where do you feel the unhealthiest?

→ Where do you need to improve your wellness the most?

→ Where does your body call out to you the most?

→ When was the last time you felt really healthy?

→ When is wellness important?

→ When has your wellness been the most compromised?

→ When do you feel the strongest?

→ When do you feel the weakest physically / mentally?

→ Why do you believe you got sick?

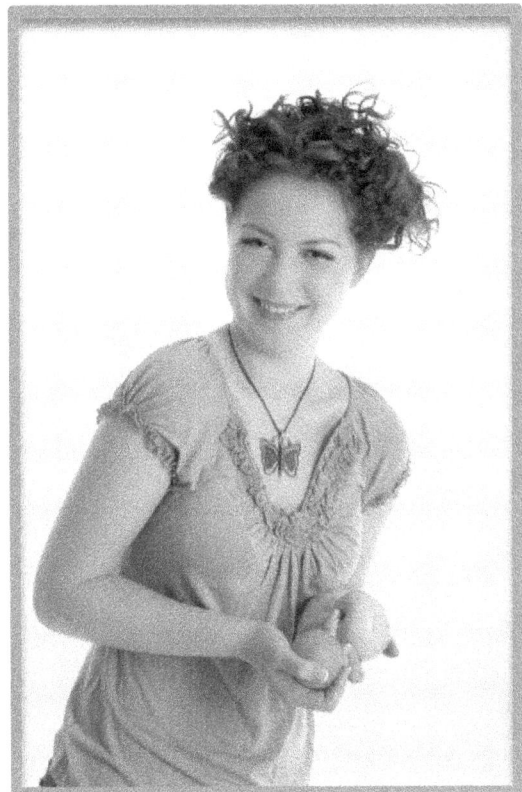

→ Why do you feel so unhealthy?

→ Why has your health become so serious?

→ How do unhealthy habits affect your overall sense of well-being?

→ How well do you sleep at night?

→ How does a good night's sleep improve your well-being?

→ How do you measure your overall health and wellness?

→ Without them saying a word, how can you tell someone is healthy?

→ How do you best recover from ill health?

→ How is healthful living learned?

→ How often do you feel on top of your game?

→ How often do you fall short?

→ How could you get the most out of your current wellness situation?

→ How much health do you think you can achieve?

→ How has your childhood / illness / stress affected your current state of wellness?

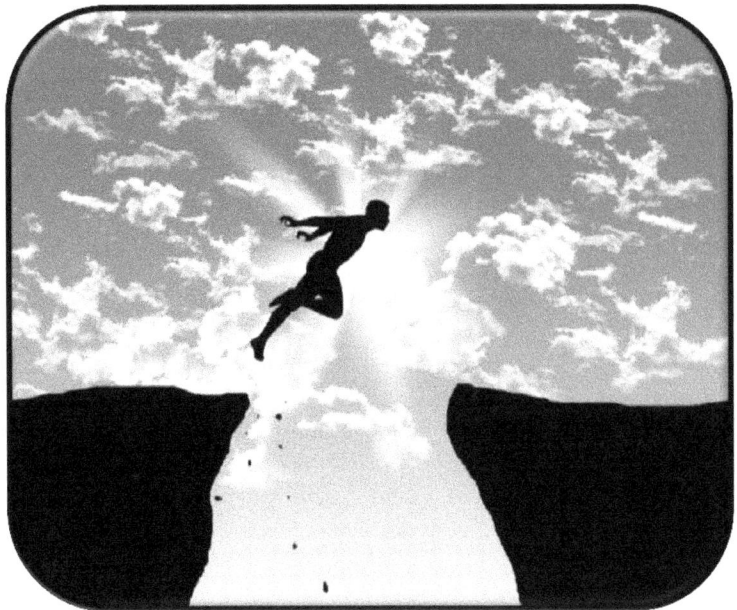

Goal Setting

Goal Setting Questions are designed to move into and forward the action. They include aspects of accountability, step-by-step action, and an understanding of what needs to be done in order to accomplish the desired goal(s).

Goal Setting Questions are intended to set the questionee up for success. In order to accomplish this there are certain factors to be considered when designing a goal plan.

SMART Goals help construct a format for creating successful goals.

Ask Goal Setting Questions when the questionee is ready to move into action.

Example of Goal Setting Questions

Questionee: I decided I want to return to college and finish my degree.

Questioner: That's great! When would you like to begin?

Questionee: Next semester but I have some things I need to do first.

Questioner: What do you see as the 1st step to take to get started?

Questionee: Well, I need to talk with an admissions counselor and figure out what credits will transfer and how many credits I need to complete my degree. Then I have to decide which classes to start with.

Questioner: That sounds like a plan. When will you make the appointment?

Questionee: This week. I am excited!
(Move onto creating SMART Goals *pg. 71)

Goal Setting Questions

→   What would it take to achieve optimal wellness?

→   What would you do if you knew you could not fail?

→   What resources are available to you that can help you achieve the wellness you seek?

→   What lifestyle changes do you need to make?

→   What lifestyle changes do you want to make?

→   What has gotten in the way?

→   What can you do to better manage stress?

→   What type of lifestyle would you like to have at 40, 50, 60, 70, etc?

→   What do you need to do now to ensure that lifestyle?

→   In what way is your current lifestyle not supporting a healthier you?

→   If your wellness didn't change, what would happen?

→   What habit would you like to break forever?

→   What new habit would you like to replace the old habit?

→   What motivates you to make the changes you need?

→   What keeps that motivation strong?

→   Where would you like your health to be in 3 months?

→   Where will having more well-being make the biggest difference?

→   When do you know that you have achieved a state of well-being?

→   When should you let go of old habits?

→ When will you know you have reached optimal wellness?

→ When would you like to achieve that?

→ Why are these goals important to you?

→ Why wouldn't you give yourself every chance to succeed?

→ Why not begin today?

→ How effective are you at maintaining healthy habits?

→ How motivated are you to make the changes you need?

→ How clear are you on what you need to change?

→ How can you fill the gaps between your ideal healthy lifestyle and where you are currently at?

→ How can changing your lifestyle serve you better?

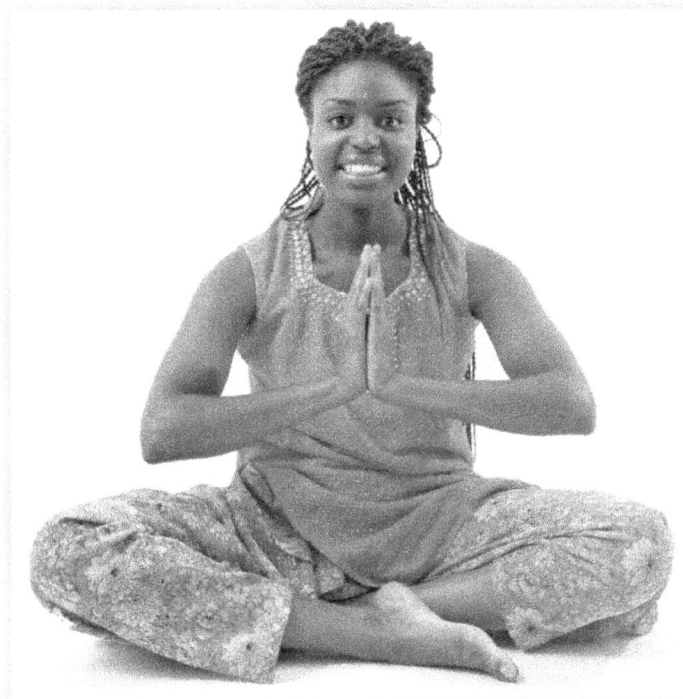

Prioritizing

Prioritizing Questions identifies and weighs importance, values and benefits. They can also be used to rank & order.

Prioritizing Questions are great to use in conjunction with Goal Setting Questions and can also help reduce overwhelm.

Ask Prioritizing Questions when the questionee needs to put their priorities in order or examine what is important to them.

Example of Prioritizing Questions

Questionee: I have so many things I need to get done. I feel overwhelmed!

Questioner: That is understandable considering all you have on your plate. Let's make a list of everything you have to do.

Questionee: OK.

(Together they create a list of to-do's)

Questionee: That's a lot! No wonder I feel overwhelmed.

Questioner: I hear you! Let's chunk it down. Of these 12 items, which are the most urgent and necessary to get done this week?

Questionee: I would have to say numbers 3, 6 and 7. The others can wait. I feel much better.

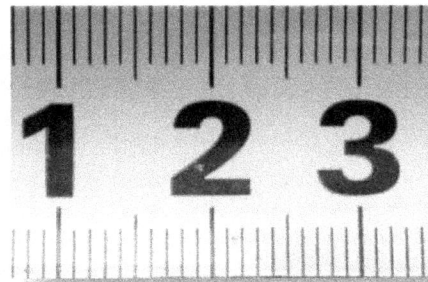

Prioritizing Questions

→ Who do you need to consider?

→ Who is your number one priority?

→ Who would you become if you placed your wellness on the top of your priority list?

→ Who supports your priorities?

→ With whom do you share your priorities?

→ What are qualities and characteristics of a healthy person?

→ What qualities do the healthiest people possess?

→ What are your top 3-5 wellness must-haves?

→ What is more important to your well-being: mind, body or spirit?

→ What needs attending to the most right now, your mind, body or spirit?

→ What is your number one priority?

→ What gets in the way of you keeping your wellness as your number one priority?

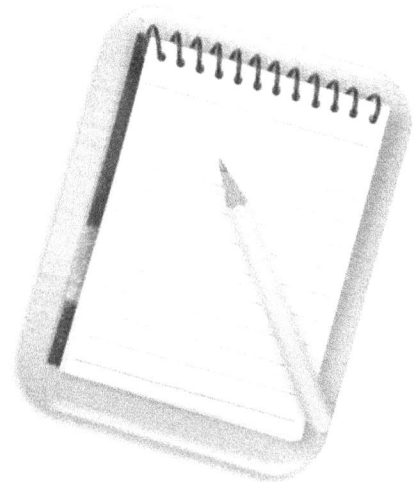

→ What can be done about that?

→ What can't you live without?

→ What are the best things you can do to meet what your body needs?

→ Where do you need to focus your efforts?

→ Where can you shift your priorities to achieve greater wellness?

→ When do you need to make that a priority?

→ When do you feel your priorities are fully in alignment with your goals?

→ When do you feel they fall short?

→ How important is it for you to feel healthy?

→ In the grand scheme of things, how important is wellness really?

→ How could you align your wellness priorities with your core values?

→ How would prioritizing your goals help you?

→ How often do you put your personal priorities aside for others?

→ How can you reclaim what is most important to you?

→ Why is your wellness important to you?

→ Why is living well important?

→ Why is it important to achieve a healthy lifestyle now?

→ Why should you adopt a healthier lifestyle?

→ Why must you heal?

→ Why is this important to you right now?

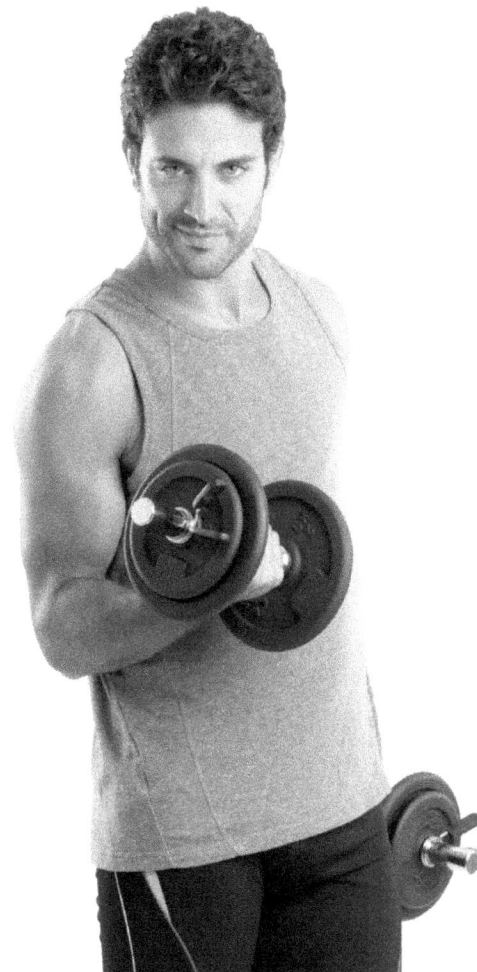

Probing

Probing Questions make the questionee go deeper, drawing out more details, concerns, challenges, knowledge, and issues about a particular situation. A good Probing Question requires thought. These questions are used to get out the root of the situation, and reveal thoughts, feelings, and details under the surface.

Ask Probing Questions when going deeper into an issue or concern will bring greater insight and help uncover new awareness; thoughts and feelings lying below the surface.

Example of Probing Questions

Questionee: I really don't want to do my presentation tomorrow.

Questioner: Why not?

Questionee: I don't know. Even though I put a lot of time into preparing it, I guess I don't think it's very good. I'd rather hold off until I can make it better.

Questioner: From what you described last time, it appears you have a solid presentation.

Questionee: Yeah, I guess so. I just think it could be better.

Questioner: Putting the presentation itself aside, what are you really worried about?

Questionee: (Pause) That I will freeze...nothing will come out of my mouth and look like a bumbling fool!

Questioner: That is quite a worry.

Questionee: I didn't realize how anxious I am about speaking to the group.

Questioner: How would it be for us to work on that together?

Questionee: Yes, please! It would be great.

Probing Questions

→ Who do you admire most for their healthy lifestyle? Why?

→ Aside from yourself, who else will be most affected by a healthier you?

→ Who has influenced your current state of wellness?

→ Who has influenced your ideas of wellness?

→ What beliefs do you have around wellness?

→ What effects do these beliefs have on your life and wellness?

→ What does stress do to your wellness?

→ In what way do your thoughts affect your overall well-being?

→ What beliefs do you have about yourself that affect your overall wellness?

→ In what way is your current lifestyle supporting a healthier you?

→ What place should spirituality have in your wellness plan?

→ If you were in your advanced years and had an opportunity to tell a youngster the most important thing you learned about living a healthy life, what you tell them?

→ If you had to describe wellness in just three words, what would you say?

→ If someone lived only from the head, what impact would that have on their overall wellness?

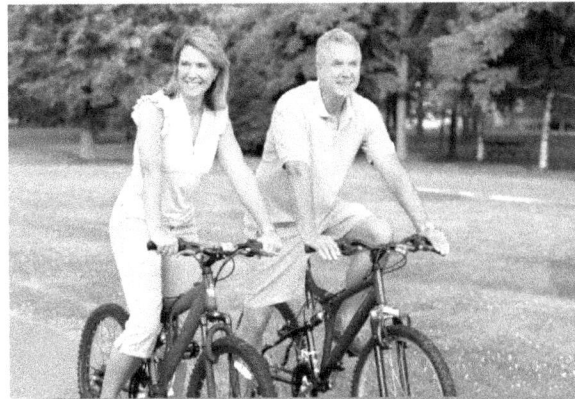

→ If someone lived only from the heart, what impact would that have on their overall wellness?

→ What would a combination of the two look like?

→ What is the one thing you must have to feel healthy?

→ Where can you use a wellness make-over?

→ Where does your strength come from?

→ Where can you beef up your wellness regime?

→ Where in your life are you feeling 100%?

→ Where might your wellness end up if you do nothing?

→ Where could you use more accountability?

→ When was your belief of what is healthy formed?

→ When have you lived healthfully in the past?

→ When was the last time you felt truly healthy?

→ Why do you place so much value on health and well-being?

→ Why have you let your health go?

→ Why are you determined to regain your wellness?

→ Why have you let your wellness plan slip away?

→ How comfortable are you letting go of unhealthy habits?

→ How does your wellness define you?

→ How does your health prevent you from being who you truly are?

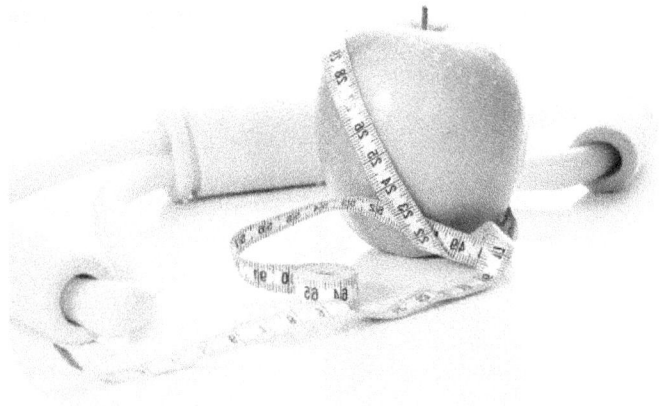

→ How can mind / body / spirit integration affect your health?

→ How well do you model wellness for others?

→ How do emotions affect your wellness?

→ How do you know when your wellness falters?

→ How has your wellness changed you?

→ How does your body talk to you?

→ Overall, how healthy do you feel?

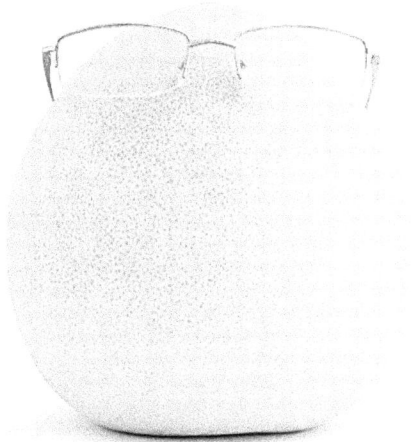

New Perspectives

New Perspective Questions are designed to shift the direction of thinking. By shifting thinking the questionee can shift the way they approach the world and situations. These questions often create "aha" moments as they elicit options and possibilities previously not considered.

Ask New Perspective Questions when the questionee persists in levels of thinking that include anger, blame, victim, trapped or when they are unable / unwilling to see alternatives.

Example of New Perspective Questions

Questionee: I think my sister is upset with me.

Questioner: What makes you think that?

Questionee: Because she hasn't returned my calls this week.

Questioner: How certain are you she is upset with you?

Questionee: Well, why else wouldn't she call me back?

Questioner: Great question! What might be some other reasons she hasn't called you back yet?

Questionee: Well, maybe she's really busy with work. I know she had a big project she was working on and her boss can set some tough deadlines. I bet that's it.

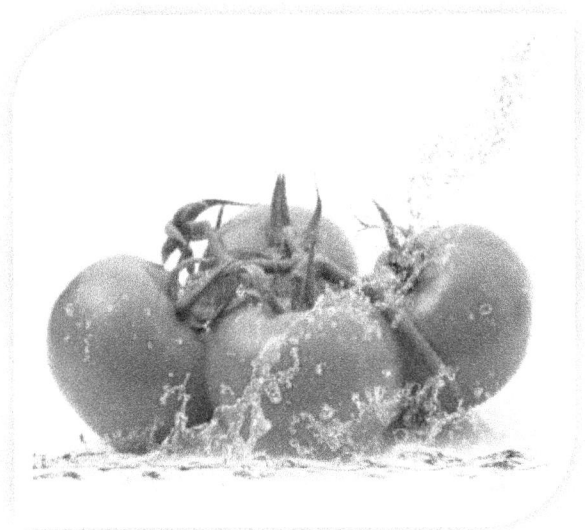

New Perspectives

→ Who are you capable of becoming?

→ Who would you be if you had optimal wellness?

→ Whose support do you need to gain for success?

→ What would be a completely different way of viewing that?

→ If your body could talk to you, what would it say?

→ What haven't you thought of yet?

→ If your wellness did a 360, what would that look like?

→ To what health warnings are you not listening?

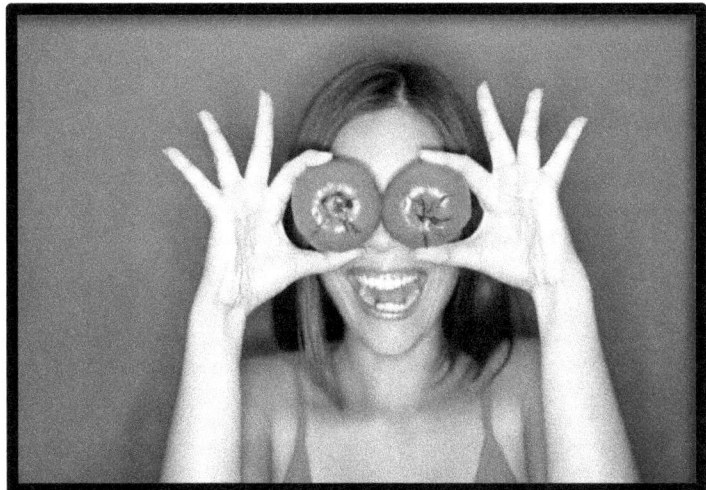

→ If your body was a store, and you were looking in through the window, what kind of store would you be?

→ What do you need to be able to put yourself first?

→ When you look in the mirror, what do you see?

→ Where have you used your body like a mean machine?

→ Where have you used your body like a robot?

→ Where have you used your body like a beast of burden?

→ Where does your body really want to go?

→ When have you taken the very best care of yourself?

→ When have you let your health go to the dogs?

→ When do you hide from what your body is trying to tell you?

→ When do you listen to what your body is trying to tell you?

→ When would it be too late to make the changes you want?

→ When have you avoided looking at yourself in the mirror?

→ Why would you let your body go?

→ Why wouldn't you consider yourself beautiful / handsome?

→ Why does your body need you?

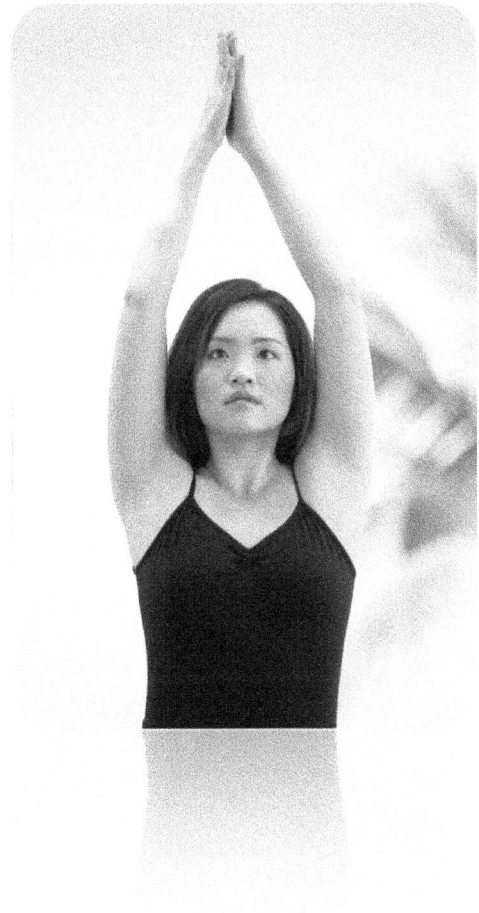

→ Why do you need your body?

→ How can you shift these thoughts to better serve you?

→ How does your health affect your wellness?

→ How can you look at exercising as play rather than work?

→ How can you address this from a place of love for yourself?

→ How much do your thoughts affect your health?

→ How would your body chew you out if it got a chance?

→ How would your body congratulate you?

→ How can your mind and body unite for the common good?

Scaling

Scaling Questions help gauge and determine the level of concern, commitment, and importance. They are a tool that identifies where the questionee would position themselves, the situation or determining a level. Scaling Questions can be used to help measure progress, attitude and behavioral change, and situational shifts.

Ask Scaling Questions when the questionee wants to gauge the level of concern, commitment, or importance of a situation or concern.

Example of Scaling Questions

Questioner: On a scale of 1-10, 1 being not at all and 10 being extremely, how important is that for you?

Questionee: I would say about an 8.5.

Questioner: That's pretty important!

Questionee: Yes, it really it.

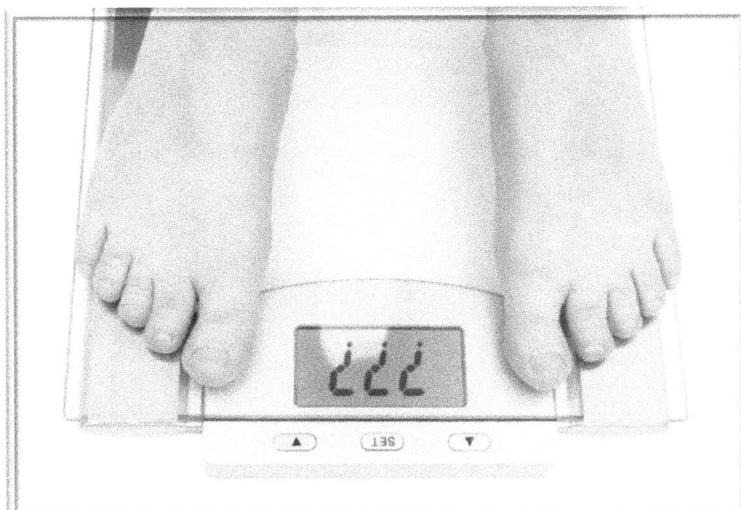

Scaling Questions

→ On a Scale of 1 to 10 (10 = completely satisfied and 1 = completely dissatisfied) where would you rank your overall health? Why did you rank yourself that way?

→ On a Scale of 1 to 10 (10 = completely and 1 = not at all) how well do you maintain a healthy lifestyle? Why did you rank yourself that way?

→ On a Scale of 1 to 10, (10 = completely and 1 = not at all), how ready are you to make the changes you need? Why did you rank yourself that way?

→ On a Scale of 1 to 10, (10 = completely and 1 = not at all), how close are you to your ideal health? Why did you rank yourself that way?

→ On a Scale of 1 to 10 (10 = completely and 1 = not at all) how ready are you to start now? Why did you rank yourself that way?

→ On a Scale of 1 to 10 (10 = completely and 1 = not at all) how easy will this transition be for you? Why did you rank yourself that way?

→ On a Scale of 1 to 10, (10 is completely and 1 is not at all) how much support do you have to help you achieve this? Why did you rank yourself that way?

→ On a Scale of 1 to 10, (10 = completely and 1 = not at all) how healthy do you feel right now? Why did you rank yourself that way?

→ On a Scale of 1 to 10, (10 = completely and 1= not at all) how much is stress a part of your unhealthy life-style? Why did you rank yourself that way?

→ On a Scale of 1 to 10 (10 = completely and 1 = not at all) how much is your body image influenced by our culture / media? Why did you rank yourself that way?

Wellness Wheel Assessment

Directions: for each section of the Wellness Wheel, circle the number that represents your current level of satisfaction in that area. The higher the number, the greater your level of satisfaction.

WELLNESS

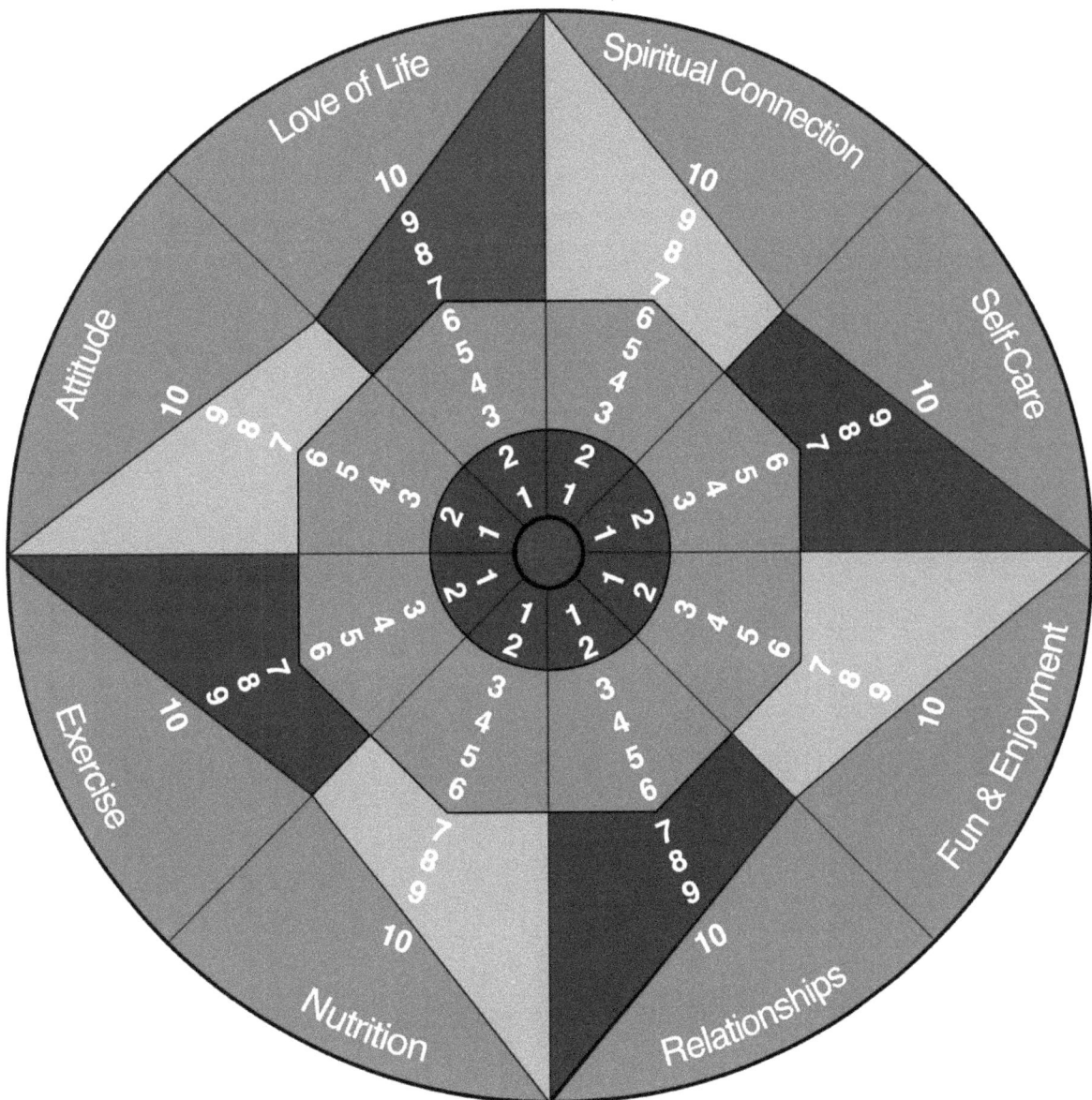

Attitude

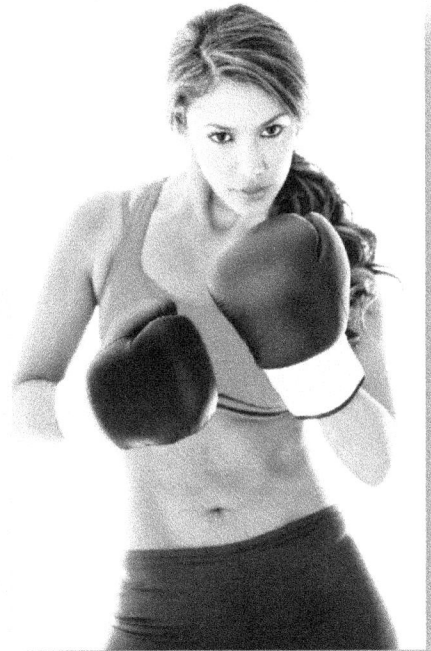

Who

→ Who would you be without an upbeat attitude?

→ Who epitomizes hopefulness to you?

→ With whom do you have the most difficult time remaining positive? Why?

→ With whom do you have the easiest time remaining positive? Why?

→ Who in your life needs your positivity most?

What

→ What does positive thinking mean to you?

→ What are the benefits of being positive about your life?

→ What is the downside?

→ What could you do to become more positive?

→ What would you do if you knew you could not fail?

Where

→ Where do you want to be more positive?

→ Where do you find yourself succumbing to negativity?

→ Where do you most need a positive attitude?

→ Where would you be if optimism was your guiding light?

→ Where can you let go of worry?

When

→ When is being positive most essential?

→ When is positive thinking a liability?

→ When would you use positive thinking to gain the best results?

→ When are you most positive? Why?

→ When are you the least? Why?

Why

→ Why is having a positive attitude important?

→ Why would changing your negative thoughts help you?

→ Why do you think you have negative thoughts?

→ Why is positive thinking beneficial?

→ Why is it hard to stay positive?

How

→ How optimistic are you?

→ How do your thoughts affect your overall wellness?

→ How will being more positive help you achieve your health-related goals?

→ How can your positive thinking be cultivated?

→ How would others benefit from your positivity?

Your Questions on Attitude

→ _____

→ _____

→ _____

→ _____

Love of Life

Who

→ Who zaps your energy? Why?

→ Who energizes you? Why?

→ Who would you be if you had all the energy in the world?

→ Who do you admire for their vitality?

→ Who helps you feel more alive?

What

→ What is vitality?

→ What needs to happen for you to feel more energized?

→ What does being fully alive mean to you?

→ What would you do if you had more energy?

→ What do you most need to let go of to feel more vital?

Where

→ Where do your life forces tend to break down for you?

→ Where is your energy weakest?

→ Where is your energy strongest?

→ Where would your health be if your vitality was super-charged?

→ Where do you want to feel stronger?

When

→ When do you feel the most depleted?

→ When do you feel the most energized?

→ When in your day are you the lowest? Why?

→ When in your life have you felt the most vital?

→ When have you felt the least vital?

Why

→ Why is vitality important to you?

→ Why do you want more vigor in your life?

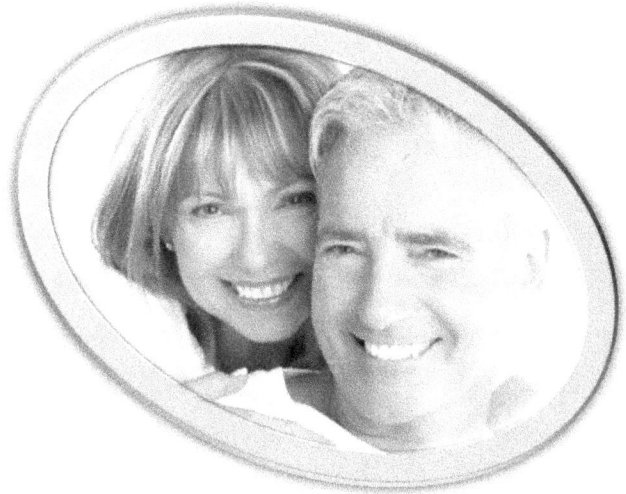

→ Why do you need to feel more alive?

→ Why is having more energy necessary?

→ Why has your vitality been hampered?

How

→ How does your current level of vitality affect your life?

→ How alive do you feel?

→ How can you begin to feel more alive?

→ How would your life & health be different if you had greater vitality?

→ How would others benefit?

Your Questions on Love of Life

→ _____

→ _____

→ _____

→ _____

Relationships

Who

→   Whose help is needed to accomplish your wellness goals?

→   Who may try to sabotage your efforts?

→   Who gives you strength?

→   Who would you like to add to your support network?

→   Who is currently a part of your support system?

What

→   What value do relationships hold for you?

→   What type of support do you need?

→   What relationships do you cherish most?

→   What type of relationship depletes you most?

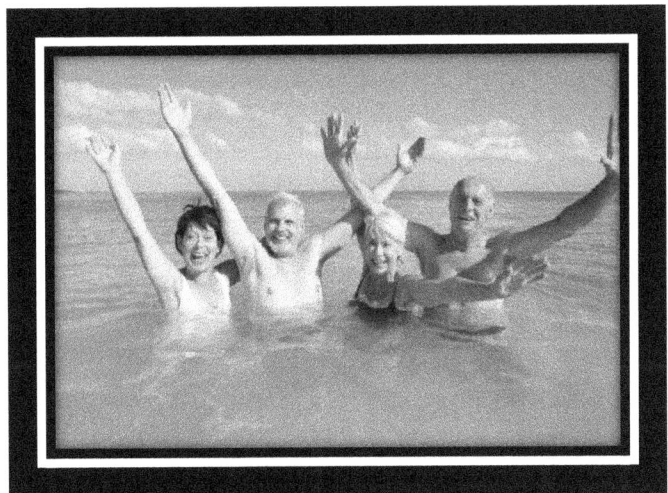

→   What type of relationship energizes you?

Where

→   Where do you feel the most connected with others?

→   Where do you feel least connected?

→   Where do you need more support?

→   Where do you still need to make changes?

→   Where are you resisting support?

When

→   When do you feel the most connected with others?

→   When do you feel the most isolated?

→   When have you been lifted up by another?

→   When have you been put down?

→   When are your relationships at their best?

Why

→   Why are healthy relationships important to you?

→   Why do you engage with people who zap your energy?

→   Why are you hoping to improve that relationship?

→   Why is asking for help hard?

→   Why would your overall sense of well-being improve by having better relationships?

How

→   How do you measure the health of your relationships?

→   How have relationships affected your health and well-being?

→   How has not having enough support affected you?

→   How can you begin to get the support you need?

→   How can you begin to cultivate healthier relationships?

Your Questions on Relationships

→   _____

→   _____

→   _____

→   _____

Spiritual Connection

Who

→   Who is your Higher Self?

→   Who would you be without access to that part of you?

→   Who do you become when fully connected spiritually?

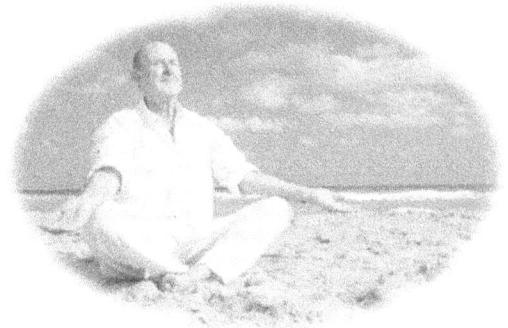

→   Who supports your spiritual strivings?

→   Who inspires you to be your best?

What

→   What needs to change?

→   What type of spiritual practice do you need?

→   What does spiritual connectedness mean to you?

→   What is the best thing about feeling connected spiritually?

→   What does your inner wisdom say about your overall well-being?

Where

→   Where is your spiritual connection the strongest?

→   Where is your spiritual connection the weakest?

→   Where do you need to feel more connection?

→   Where are you avoiding connecting spiritually?

→   Where are you resisting your inner guidance?

When

→   When has your spiritual connectedness been at its best?

→   When has it been at its worst?

→ When are you best able to listen for inner guidance?

→ When do you set time aside for your spiritual practice?

→ When is the best time to call on your Higher Power?

Why

→ Why is having a connection to your Higher Power important?

→ Why have you tried to go it alone?

→ Why do you need a deep sense of connection?

→ Why would having a stronger connection with your Higher Power help you?

→ Why is asking for help hard?

How

→ How does having a strong spiritual connection help you achieve your wellness goals?

→ How willing are you to engage in regular spiritual practice?

→ How would this help your overall well-being?

→ How often do you seek spiritual connection?

→ How can you begin to build a stronger connection with your Higher Power?

Your Questions on Spiritual Connection

→ _____

→ _____

→ _____

→ _____

→ _____

Fun & Enjoyment

Who

→   With whom do you like to do things?

→   With whom would you like to do more things?

→   Who enjoys spending time with you?

→   With whom do you like to spend time?

→   With whom do you have the most fun?

What

→   What is enjoyable to you?

→   What activities do you naturally gravitate towards?

→   What would you like to do that you haven't yet?

→   What is one activity you could make more enjoyable?

→   In what new activity would you most like to engage?

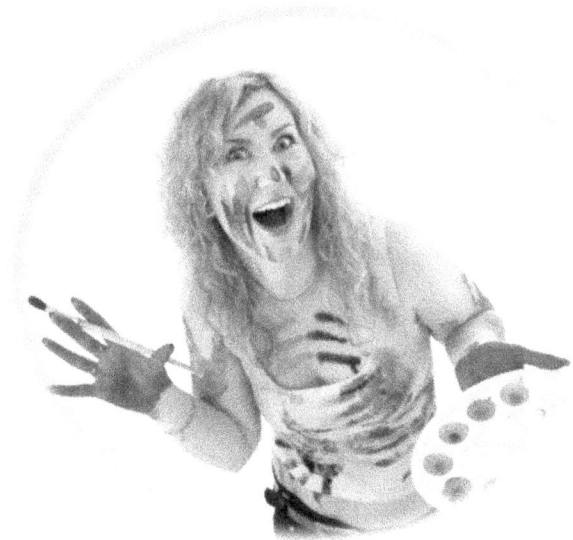

Where

→   Where do you most enjoy spending time?

→   Where would you like to go?

→   Where do you need more enjoyment in life?

→   Where has the fun gone out?

→   Where could you stretch yourself to enjoy life more?

When

→ When do you enjoy life most?

→ When do you enjoy life least?

→ When is the best time for you to get away?

→ When would you like to do that?

→ When have you had the most fun?

Why

→ Why are having enjoyable activities important to you?

→ Why have you stopped that particular activity?

→ Why would you feel better if you engaged in more enjoyable activities?

→ Why do you like to be active?

→ Why is having fun important to your well-being?

How

→ How do you feel about your current activities?

→ How would you & your wellness benefit from having more fun?

→ How would those around you benefit?

→ How can you begin to engage in more enjoyable activities?

→ How many of your current activities are draining you?

Your Questions on Fun & Enjoyment

→ _____

→ _____

→ _____

→ _____

Self-Care

Who

→ Who supports you taking good care of yourself?

→ Who sabotages your efforts? How?

→ To whom can you delegate? How?

→ Who epitomizes excellent self-care?

→ Who would you be if you took really good care of yourself all the time?

What

→ What does self-care mean to you?

→ What are your current self-care practices?

→ In what way(s) do you need to take better care of yourself?

→ What gets in your way?

→ What do you most need to let go of?

Where

→ Where do you relax the most?

→ Where do you need to take better care of yourself?

→ Where will you be in 3 months if you continue down this path?

→ Where do you need to de-stress?

→ Where are you the most at peace?

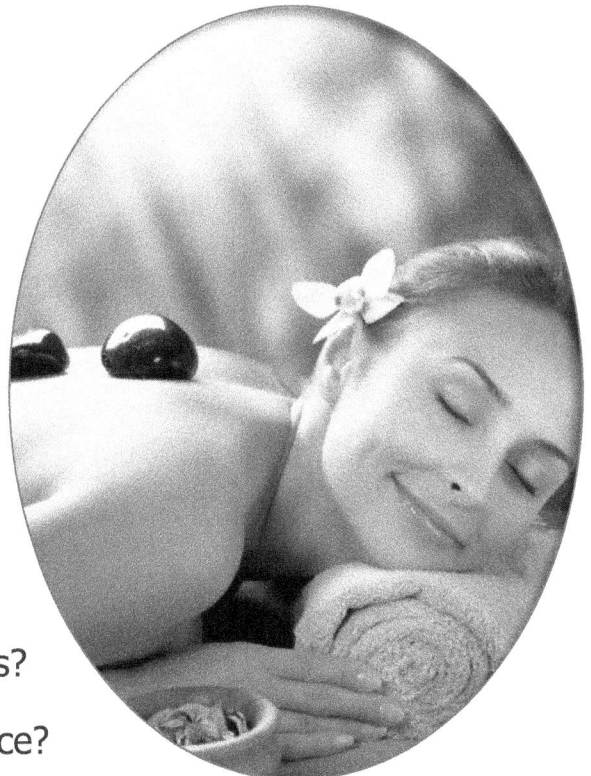

When

→ When do you need time apart?

→ When do you take the best care of yourself?

→ When do you beat yourself down?

→ When have you been able to practice excellent self-care most successfully?

→ When have you felt the most cared for?

Why

→ Why is taking good care of yourself important?

→ Why has it been hard to take good care of yourself in the past?

→ Why do you push yourself so hard?

→ Why do you usually put others first?

→ Why are the needs of others more important than your own?

How

→ How are self-care and overall well-being related?

→ How do you take care of yourself now?

→ How would you like to take better care of yourself?

→ How open are you to receiving help from others?

→ How often to you put yourself first?

Your Questions on Self-Care

→ _____

→ _____

→ _____

→ _____

Nutrition

Who

→ Who supports your eating well? Why?

→ Who sabotages your efforts? How?

→ Who is a good role model for healthy eating? In what way?

→ Who can help you achieve your goals? How?

→ Who has most influenced your eating habits? How?

What

→ What does nutrition mean to you?

→ What is important about understanding how your emotions affect your eating?

→ What are your beliefs about healthy eating?

→ What is the hardest non-nutritious food to let go of? Why?

→ What do you most want to change about the way you eat?

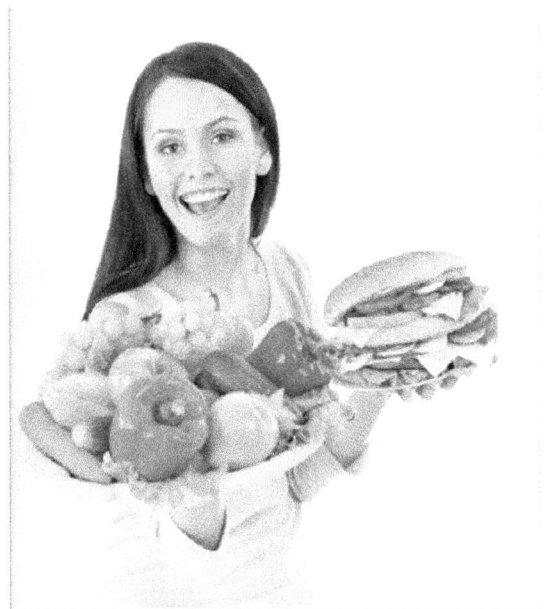

Where

→ Where are your eating habits the healthiest?

→ Where are your eating habits the worst?

→ Where would you be if you successfully adopted a healthy diet?

→ Where will you be if you don't?

→ Where do your convictions break down?

When

→ When are you most aware of how your emotions influence how you eat?

→ When are you least aware?

→ When is sticking to a healthy eating plan the easiest for you?

→ When is it the hardest?

→ When would you like to begin changing your eating habits for good?

Why

→ Why is eating well important to you?

→ Why do you eat things that are bad for you?

→ Why do you enjoy nutritious foods?

→ Why would changing your eating habits help you?

→ Why have you had a hard time sticking to a healthy diet?

How

→ How does your current diet help you?

→ How does your current diet harm you?

→ How could you begin to change that?

→ How do emotions influence your eating choices?

→ How would eating nutritiously help you achieve other goals?

Your Questions on Nutrition

→ _____

→ _____

→ _____

→ _____

Exercise

Who

→ Who would you be if you reached your ideal?

→ Who do you admire for their dedication to physically fitness?

→ Who motivates you to stay in shape?

→ Who would you become without a solid mind-body plan?

→ Who can help you achieve your fitness goals?

What

→ What would be an ideal exercise plan for you?

→ What type of physical activity to you like best?

→ What does being physically fit mean to you?

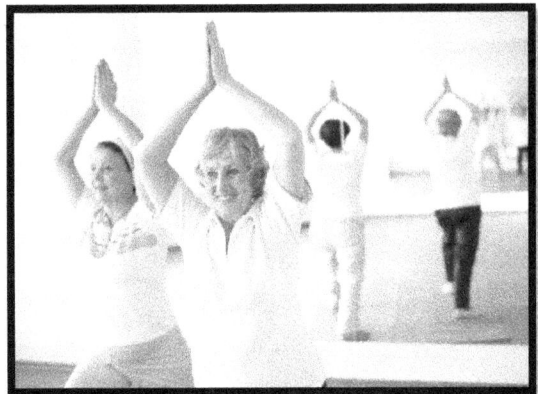

→ What blocks your ability to stick with your exercise plan?

→ What does your body need to feel healthier?

Where

→ Where do you like to exercise?

→ Where does your exercise regime break down?

→ Where will you be in 3 months if you don't change your level of physical activity?

→ Where would you like your exercise to be in 3 months?

→ Where has a mind-body exercise plan been the easiest for you to maintain?

When

→ When do you like to exercise?

→ When do you dislike exercising?

→ When have you been the most disciplined? The least?

→ When do you most need physical activity?

→ When are you the least likely to stay with your plan?

Why

→ Why do you like to exercise?

→ Why would having a disciplined physical practice help you?

→ Why do you need to feel more in your body?

→ Why have you struggled with your exercise regime in the past?

→ Why do you want to change your current level of physical activity?

How

→ How do you feel about regular exercise?

→ How have you succeeded in the past with maintaining a good exercise plan?

→ How important is having a healthy body?

→ How does a lack of time affect your ability to attend to your body's needs?

→ How often would you like to get physically active?

Your Questions on Exercise

→ _____

→ _____

→ _____

Wellness Values Assessment

Directions: Identify your top 8 Health & Wellness Values / Qualities. How closely do you live these Values / Qualities?

☐ Abundance	
☐ Acceptance	☐ Efficiency
☐ Accountability	☐ Empowered
☐ Achievement	☐ Encouragement
☐ Action	☐ Endurance
☐ Active	☐ Energy
☐ Activity	☐ Enjoyment
☐ Adaptability	☐ Enthusiasm
☐ Aliveness	☐ Fitness
☐ Assertiveness	☐ Flexibility
☐ Authenticity	☐ Focus
☐ Awareness	☐ Follow-Through
☐ Balance	☐ Free Will
☐ Beauty	☐ Freedom
☐ Being	☐ Fulfillment
☐ Can Do Attitude	☐ Fun
☐ Change	☐ Goal-Oriented
☐ Cheerfulness	☐ Gratitude
☐ Comfort	☐ Growth
☐ Commitment	☐ Healing
☐ Concentration	☐ Health
☐ Connectedness	☐ Healthy Relationships
☐ Consciousness	☐ Higher Power
☐ Courage	☐ Honesty
☐ Dedication	☐ Humor
☐ Desire	☐ Imagination
☐ Diet	☐ Inspiration
☐ Disciplined	☐ Intention

☐ Intuition	☐ Self-Knowledge
☐ Letting Go	☐ Self-Realization
☐ Life	☐ Setting Boundaries
☐ Love	☐ Silence
☐ Meditation	☐ Simplicity
☐ Mindfulness	☐ Spirit
☐ Motivation	☐ Spirituality
☐ Mutual Support	☐ Spontaneity
☐ Non-judgment	☐ Stamina
☐ Non-resistance	☐ Steadfastness
☐ Nutrition	☐ Stillness
☐ Optimistic	☐ Strength
☐ Order	☐ Structure
☐ Passion	☐ Support
☐ Patience	☐ Surrender
☐ Peace	☐ Synergy
☐ Physicality	☐ Transformation
☐ Playfulness	☐ Trust
☐ Positive Thinking	☐ Understanding
☐ Potential	☐ Vigor
☐ Power	☐ Visualization
☐ Pro-Active	☐ Vitality
☐ Purifying	☐ Well-being
☐ Relaxation	☐ Wellness
☐ Release	☐ Wholeness
☐ Rest	☐ Will
☐ Rigor	☐ Win-Win Attitude
☐ Robustness	☐ Wisdom
☐ Self-Authority	☐ Zeal
☐ Self-Awareness	☐ _____
☐ Self-Care	☐ _____
☐ Self-Esteem	☐ _____
☐ Self-Growth	

Blank Wellness Wheel

Directions: In the blank sections of the wheel add your top 8 Wellness Values / Qualities from the previous assessment. For each section, circle the number that represents your current level of satisfaction in that area. The higher the number, the greater your level of satisfaction.

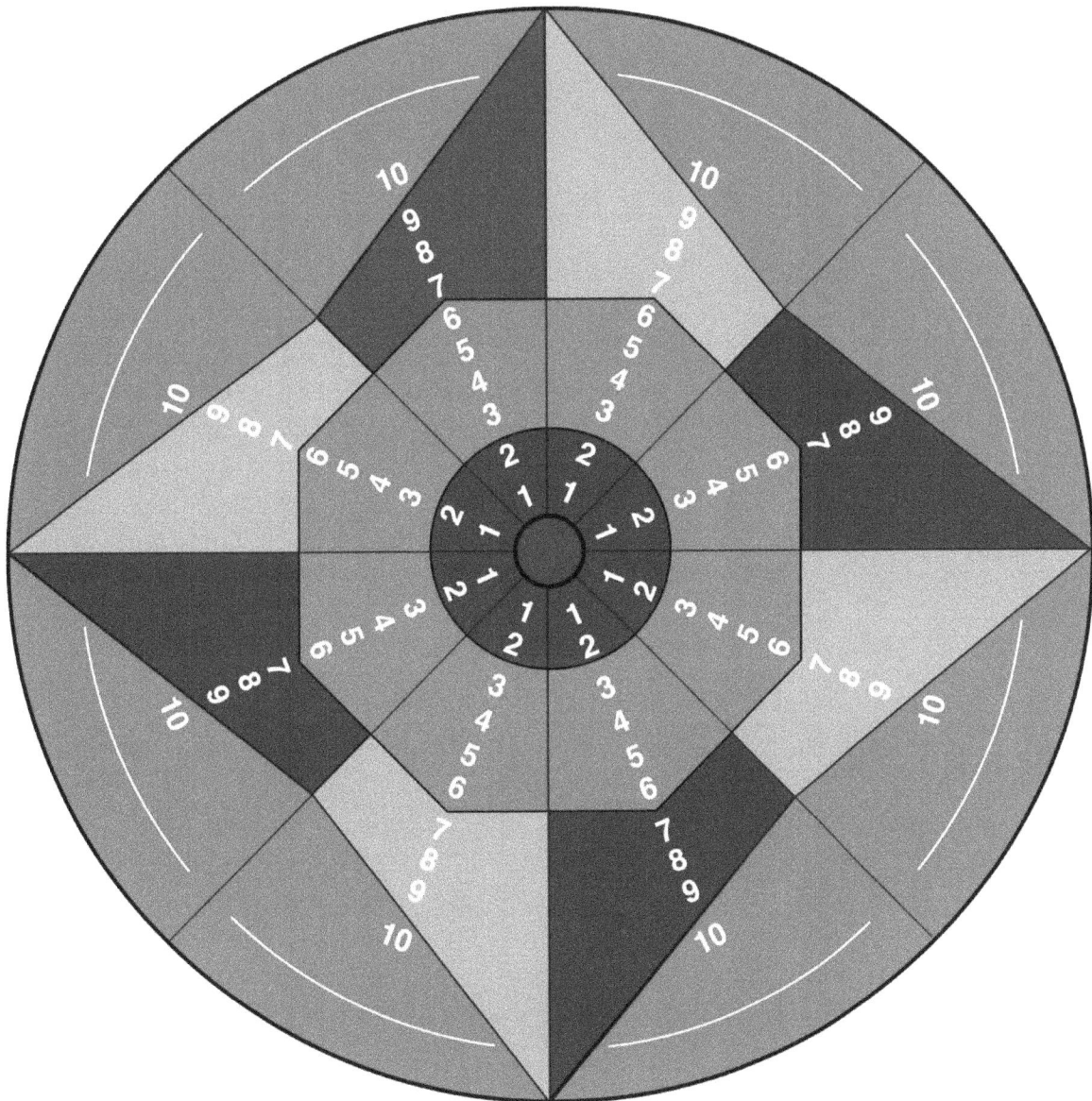

Wellness Quotes

The greatest wealth is health.
~ Virgil

Take care of your body. It's the only place you have to live.
~ Jim Rohn

If it is to be, it is up to me.
~ Anon

Your body is a temple, but only if you treat it as one.
~ Astrid Alauda

A harmonious relationship with one you love can enhance your work, health and entire well-being.
~ Doc Childe

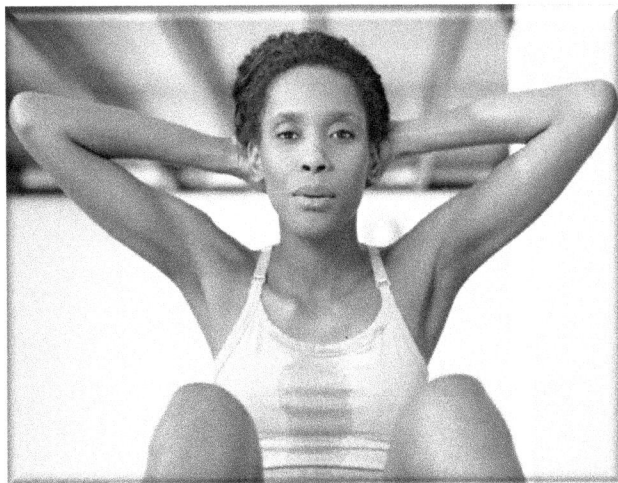

Quit worrying about your health. It'll go away.
~ Robert Orbin

Love cures people — both the ones who give it and the ones who receive it.
~ Dr. Karl Menninger

No pressure, no diamonds.
~ Mary Case

I don't want to be a passenger in my own life.
~ Diane Ackerman

Time and health are two precious assets that we don't recognize and appreciate until they have been depleted.
~ Denis Waitley

Attitude is a little thing that makes a big difference.
~ Winston Churchill

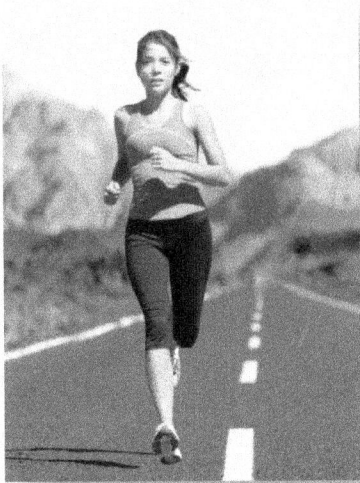

To keep the body in good health is a duty... otherwise we shall not be able to keep our mind strong and clear.
~ Buddha

When man is serene, the pulse of the heart flows and connects, just as pearls are joined together or like a string of red jade, then one can talk about a healthy heart.
~ The Yellow Emperor's Canon of Internal Medicine, 2500 B.C.

Fitness - if it came in a bottle, everybody would have a great body.
~ Cher

A sad soul can kill you quicker than a germ.
~ John Steinbeck

To get rich never risk your health. For it is the truth that health is the wealth of wealth.
~ Richard Baker

The world belongs to the energetic.
~ Ralph Waldo Emerson

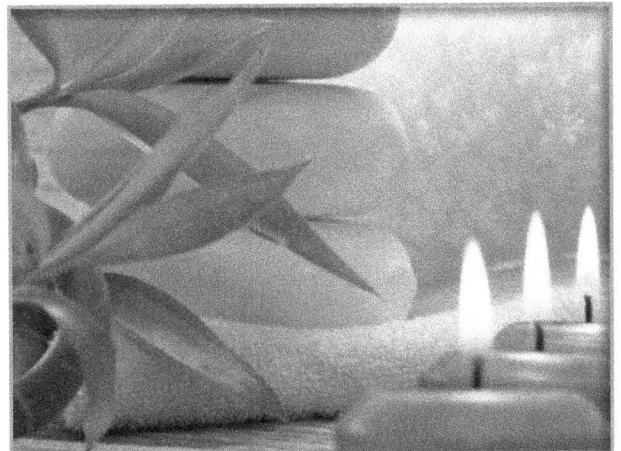

Life expectancy would grow by leaps and bounds if green vegetables smelled as good as bacon.
~ Doug Larson

It's so hard when I have to, and so easy when I want to.
> ~ Annie Gottlier

If your thoughts are thoughts that draw low-frequency energy current to you, your physical and emotional attitudes will deteriorate, and emotional or physical disease will follow, whereas thoughts that draw high-frequency energy current to you create physical and emotional health.
> ~ Gary Zukav

The groundwork of all happiness is health.
> ~ Leigh Hunt

Movement is a medicine for creating change in a person's physical, emotional, and mental states.
> ~ Carol Welch

He who has health has hope; and he who has hope has everything.
> ~ Arabian Proverb

If you don't like something, change it; if you can't change it, change the way you think about it.
> ~ Mary Engelbreit

A wise man should consider that health is the greatest of human blessings, and learn how by his own thought to derive benefit from his illnesses.
> ~ Hippocrates

He who takes medicine and neglects to diet wastes the skill of his doctors.
> ~ Chinese Proverb

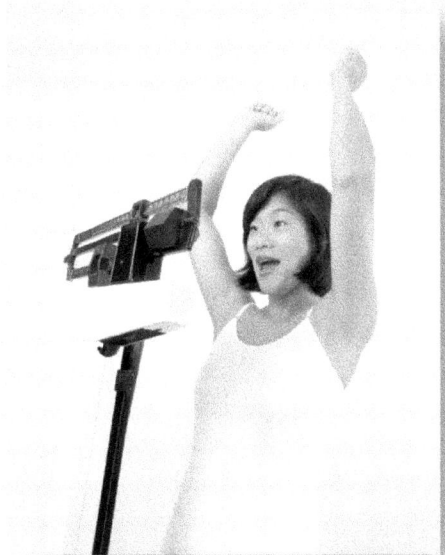

Lack of activity destroys the good condition of every human being, while movement and methodical physical exercise save it and preserve it.
~ Plato

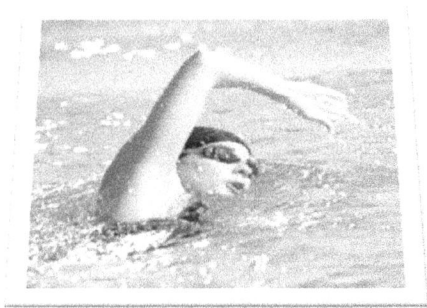

Our own physical body possesses a wisdom which we who inhabit the body lack. We give it orders which make no sense.
~ Henry Miller

As I see it, every day you do one of two things: build health or produce disease in yourself.
~ Adelle Davis

The sovereign invigorator of the body is exercise, and of all the exercises walking is the best.
~ Thomas Jefferson

Our bodies are our gardens - our wills are our gardeners.
~ William Shakespeare

I have to exercise in the morning before my brain figures out what I'm doing.
~ Marsha Doble

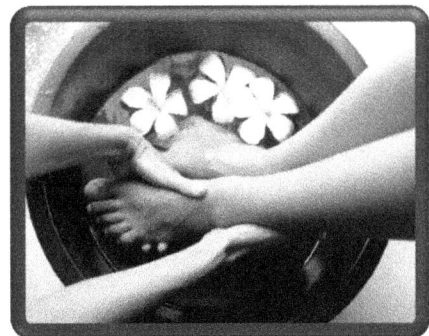

The higher your energy level, the more efficient your body. The more efficient your body, the better you feel and the more you will use your talent to produce outstanding results.
~ Anthony Robbins

People say that losing weight is no walk in the park. When I hear that I think, yeah, that's the problem.
~ Chris Adams

When health is absent, wisdom cannot reveal itself, art cannot manifest, strength cannot fight, wealth becomes useless, and intelligence cannot be applied.
~ Herophilus

If the body be feeble, the mind will not be strong.
~ Thomas Jefferson

It is amazing how much crisper the general experience of life becomes when your body is given a chance to develop a little strength.
~ Frank Duff

If your inner energy is misdirected, so will your whole life be.
~ C. Astrid Weber

Take rest; a field that has rested gives a bountiful crop.
~ Ovid

Those who think they have not time for bodily exercise will sooner or later have to find time for illness.
~ Edward Stanley

For fast-acting relief, try slowing down.
~ Lily Tomlin

The body never lies.
~ Martha Graham

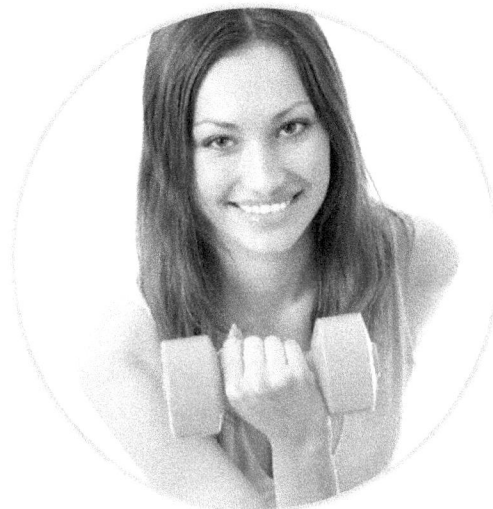

S.M.A.R.T. Goals Checklist

Specific
- ☐ What precisely is expected?
- ☐ Be as specific as possible.
- ☐ What will you have when the specific task is complete?
- ☐ What will the outcome be?

Measurable
- ☐ How would you know you have achieved success?
- ☐ How many tasks do you need to do?
- ☐ For how long?
- ☐ Make it a tangible process.

Achievable
- ☐ Is this achievable?
- ☐ What would be achievable?
- ☐ Do you have the skills or resources necessary to meet this goal?

Reasonable
- ☐ Is this a reasonable goal?
- ☐ What might be the obstacles?
- ☐ Considering everything else you have going on, can you achieve this goal?

Time-Oriented
- ☐ When will you be done?
- ☐ When will your tasks be scheduled?
- ☐ How long will it take to accomplish each task?
- ☐ When is the ideal time for this goal to be completed?

About the Work

We live in a time of great change. Faced with some of the most difficult challenges our world has ever known, we feel an urgency to find solutions to make our lives better. We want answers and we want them now!

In general, we focus on **getting the right answer not on asking the right questions.** Why is this? Perhaps it stems from an innate curiosity and a desire to make sense of the world. Perhaps it comes from a fear of the unknown or the need for a quick fix. It may also result from the need for blind acceptance of some *truth* where any form of questioning is strongly discouraged or denied. Perhaps we think we already have the answer, so why ask any questions at all? Whatever the case, there is no doubt human beings like answers.

When we focus on "getting the right answers," rather than "asking the right questions," we limit ourselves. We move into dualistic thinking: "I either have the right answer or I don't." We think in terms of yes or no, right or wrong, good or bad. **This black and white framework enables only surface inquiry**, at best, and quells deeper investigation and the ability to engage with others in meaningful ways. We lose the opportunity to generate new solutions to old problems.

Why are asking the right questions important? Because they generate beneficial lasting change. Empowering questions make possible diverse perspectives, which in turn lead to sustainable solutions to complicated challenges. They enable people to engage in dynamic transformational conversations out of which new ideas are born.

To generate the type of change our world needs, **we must raise penetrative questions to challenge current assumptions**; assumptions that keep us disempowered to affect change. The key in creating a positive, empowering future is asking positive, empowering questions now! So, what are you waiting for?

About the Authors

Kathy Jo Slusher, PCC, ELI-MP, Founder of Marketing Tao, LLC, has dedicated her life to help service-based socially conscious business owners make their business a success through sharing their passion. She believes that when your intention is on your passion and helping others, money is a natural bi-product. *It's not what you sell but what you stand for that makes you a success.* She is deeply committed to helping soloprofessionals and small business owners implement mindful marketing techniques and strategies to attract their ideal clients while making a difference in the world.

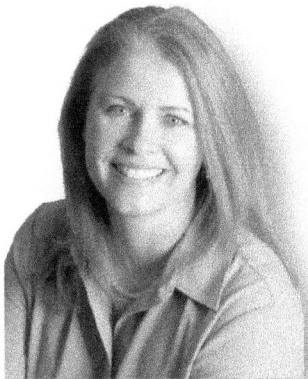

Kathy Jo is a Co-Founder of The REAL Results Coaching Exchange, partner in Coaching Skills for Leaders, a member of the International Coach Federation, and Vice-President of the United Nations Association of the US, Indianapolis Chapter.

Denny Balish, PCC, ELI-MP, Professional Certified Coach and Founder of ThreeFold Life Coaching, has dedicated her life's work to the development of Human Potential. She believes that each person has within themselves the desire and ability to be a positive force for change in the world and, by sharing one's unique gifts and talents with others, global change is possible. Denny is deeply committed to helping people and organizations get and stay powerfully on-purpose so they can be the change they wish to see in the world. Denny is a member of the International Coach Federation (ICF), Association for Global New Thought (AGNT), and founding board member of Spirit's Light Foundation, an alternative youth and family ministry with the Association of Unity Churches International.

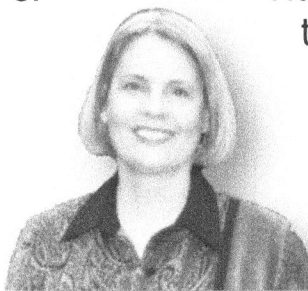

Other Valuable Resources

For Coaches, Consultants, and Service-Based Small Businesses

Ultimate Questions Books

The real power in transformation is not in the answers, but in the questions we ask. If coaches, therapists or consultants are unsure of the questions to ask, client results are greatly impacted.

This series of books is specifically designed for coaches, consultants, therapists and others who are in a place where they need some fresh ideas to get themselves, a client, or anyone else unstuck. www.UltimateQuestionsBook.com

Marketing Made Practical

Marketing Made Practical is a Home Study Program designed for those who are overwhelmed with all the options and don't have a handle on how to make the marketing process into an effective, successful strategy.

Marketing Made Practical is specifically designed for service-based soloprofessionals or small business owners who are just getting started or have a limited experience and need an organized approach to marketing. www.MarketingMadePractical.com

Marketing Strategies University

Marketing Strategies University is an online training program that walks you through how to create a strong marketing and business development plan.

Marketing Strategies University cuts to the chase of marketing. We don't dive into the theory of marketing – but focus on practical steps to create and implement powerful marketing strategies.

This unique online training program is designed for service-based soloprofessionals or small business owners who have reached a certain level in their business where they are ready to create the systems and strategies for their marketing to take them to the next level of success. www.MarketingStrategiesUniversity.com

Marketing Strategies Success

Marketing Strategies Success is an online membership forum which brings together motivation and information into a community of like-minded business owners all working to create change through their business.

Through topic specific open Q & A calls & recordings, to an interactive forum where members share ideas, to a mentoring component of Success Stories, where successful entrepreneurs share their success secrets, this group will help those who have a message to share through their business but need marketing know-how & structure to accomplish their mission. www.MarketingStrategiesSuccess.com

For Leadership Development Support

Coaching Skills for Leaders

Employees don't leave companies, they leave managers.

According to the Gallup Poll, 71% of employees studied said they were either not engaged or actively disengaged at work. This employee disengagement results in $370 Billion lost annually. That's a huge amount.

In today's environment, talented individuals are arguably an organization's most valuable resource. Yet studies show, high potential employees have a higher turnover rate than any other employee population.

Leaders need to be flexible, adaptable, creative and resourceful to deal with the reality of our economic times. Coaching Skills for Leaders will take you

and your organization through The Coaching Clinic, a specialized training program where you acquire a new approach to old issues. This process offers a step-by-step process of a coaching conversation in how to conduct & lead those difficult conversations. You will learn how to address organizational challenges through a step-by-step structured approach to facilitate your own coaching conversation, and develop partners and accountability standards across the board. Thus you will be transforming managers into true Leaders. www.Coaching-Skills-for-Leaders.com

Lifestyle, Leadership, Legacy

What are you working for?

As a business owner or executive you've worked hard to get where you are at. But how has this helped the lifestyle you want to lead? If you're tired to living to work instead of working to live, this program is for you.

We will identify your desired lifestyle, look at how to improve your leadership ability so you can more effectively lead those around you as well as your own life and create a lasting legacy to leave behind.

On-Purpose Leadership Development

For on-purpose professionals who want to develop their leadership acumen while expanding their consciousness. This program formulates a plan of action to break through all obstacles limiting your success, while building powerful skills to help you lead with purpose, including: manage conflict and chaos with greater ease, use your intuition for effortless decision-making, communicate effectively and persuasively, maximize your ability to engage and influence people in positive ways, and feel empowered to affect change in yourself and others.

For Specialized Support for Non-Profits, Social Enterprises and Cultural Creatives

Life Purpose Coaching

Empowering individuals in their midlife years to create a life of deeper meaning and purpose by not only connecting with their authentic voice and innate wisdom, but also by helping them aligning their skills, talents and interests with their desire to give back in meaningful ways.

On-Purpose Career Transition

For individuals in all phases of career and job transition who seek to purposefully align their skills and abilities with their passion for a satisfying career; one that enables them to give back in meaningful ways. Make a living while making a difference! This program is customized to fit individual needs.

For More Information Contact:

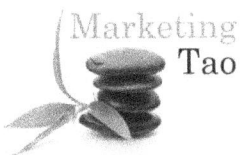

Marketing Tao, LLC
Kathy Jo Slusher
Email   info@MarketingTao.com
Call   317.536.5544
Click   www.MarketingTao.com
Click   www.TheREALResultsCoachingExchange.com

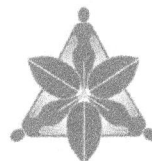

Threefold Life
Denny Balish
Email   info@threefoldlife.com
Call   708.209.6977
Click   www.Threefoldlife.com

www.ingramcontent.com/pod-product-compliance
Lightning Source LLC
Chambersburg PA
CBHW080615270326
41928CB00016B/3070